ELAINE Z HAUSER
720 BLAIR CT #H
SUNNYVALE, CA 94087

Dr. Mandell's
5•Day Allergy Relief System

Dr. Mandell's 5·Day Allergy Relief System

By Marshall Mandell, M.D.
and Lynne Waller Scanlon

THOMAS Y. CROWELL, PUBLISHERS

New York   Established 1834

Grateful acknowledgment is made for permission to reprint:

Excerpts from *Clinical Ecology*, edited by Lawrence D. Dickey, M.D., F.P.A.C. (1976). Courtesy of Charles C. Thomas, Publisher, Springfield, Illinois.

Designed by C. Linda Dingler

Library of Congress Cataloging in Publication Data

Mandell, Marshall.
    Dr. Mandell's 5-Day allergy relief system.
    1. Allergy. 2. Allergy—Prevention. I. Scanlon, Lynne Waller, joint author. II. Title. III. Title: 5-Day allergy relief system. [DNLM: 1. Hypersensitivity—Therapy—Popular works. WD300 M271d]
RC584.M34 1978   616.9'7   78-3309
ISBN 0-690-01471-6

---

79 80 81 82 83 10 9 8 7 6 5 4 3 2

Dedication

To my parents, my children and my grandchildren.

To those whom I love and to those who love me.

To my friends, office staff, and patients who believe in me and my work, and have given encouragement and comfort by their loyal support.

To those who have suffered without hope, and need wait no longer.

To my teachers, colleagues and students in bio-ecologic medicine.

To the open-minded healers of the present and future who will someday join my colleagues and me, adding their personal contributions to ours.

From all of us who are deeply committed to the study and to the treatment of human disorders caused by allergy to the natural and synthetic factors in the environment, our heartfelt thanks to you, Dr. Theron Randolph, for showing us the way. Through your efforts, each of us has a greater understanding of physical, mental, and psychosomatic illness. Through your genius, we have all become much more effective members of the healing arts.

Contents

Foreword

Abram Hoffer, M.D., Ph.D.

Dr. Marshall Mandell is one of the pioneer bio-ecologic physicians. He has shown that every tissue and organ of the body can react adversely to contact with a large variety of chemicals within our environment. Every chemical, whether it impinges on our skin, is inhaled through our lungs, or is ingested into our gastrointestinal system, can elicit these adverse reactions. This also applies to the central nervous system.

It is very difficult for physicians, especially psychiatrists, to believe that any kind of metabolic disorder, including allergic reactions, can cause syndromes which are identical with every known psychiatric disease. I am sympathetic with their plight as I have had the same difficulty. I was aware of Dr. T. Randolph's work for a couple of decades, but my interest remained academic as I concentrated practically entirely on a nutrient approach, using vitamin and mineral supplements in optimum doses. Optimum doses for many meant large doses, popularly known as "megavitamin" therapy. But many, chronic schizophrenics especially, did not respond to my best effort, using every modern approach such as drugs, electroconvulsive therapy, nutrition, supplements, in or out of hospital, with or without psychotherapy.

Over the years I began to accumulate a substantial number of chronic patients who had not responded adequately. They did not recover. About five years ago I became more and more

DR. HOFFER is editor of the *Journal of Orthomolecular Psychiatry*; President of the Huxley Institute for BioSocial Research.

concerned about this group. I became aware of the work being
done by Dr. Mandell and by Dr. William H. Philpott, an orthomolecular psychiatrist. I saw a film Dr. Mandell had made
at one of our meetings. My interest gradually arose. What de-
terred me was that I knew so little about allergies and how they
were investigated. Eventually I was forced to become involved
by my patients. A sixteen-year-old schizophrenic girl had not
responded to any treatment given her by her first psychiatrist,
then by me. One day I realized that nothing was working and
she was doomed to become a chronic, hopelessly ill schizophrenic. This realization motivated me to act. I persuaded her to fast
for four days. On the fourth day she was normal. This I had
never seen in over twenty years of practice. She was allergic to
milk and a number of other foods. A glass of milk reactivated
her psychosis in an hour. Over the next two years I made about
160 patients fast. About 100 responded in the same way. This
work has been corroborated by other orthomolecular psychiatrists. There is no further doubt in my mind that certain people's brains react adversely to a variety of substances by becoming schizophrenic. If cerebral allergy can cause that most
deadly of all mental diseases—schizophrenia—it can surely
mimic all the other conditions as well, such as learning and
behavior disorders, depression, anxiety, etc., and it does.

I am very grateful to Dr. Mandell because his work and his
enthusiasm and interest in sharing his knowledge with others
has allowed me to cure a large number of psychiatric patients
who otherwise would still be ill.

The message in this book is immensely important for every
person who has anything to do with people who are sick. For
every illness may have an allergic basis or component which
will require special attention to what Dr. Mandell calls "bio-
ecology." He and his co-workers in this field have made an
incalculable contribution to every aspect of medicine, including psychiatry.

Preface

Theron G. Randolph, M.D.,
F.A.C.A., F.A.A.A., A.A.C.P.

Many intelligent citizens are tired of being chronically ill for
no apparent reason. Of those who have consulted physicians,
some are unhappy because they cannot accept their doctor's
reassurance that there is nothing wrong with them. Others are
not pleased to have their symptoms treated by drugs, still without knowing why they are sick. Those who find themselves in
this fix, that is, having an untreated or unsatisfactorily treated
chronic illness, will profit by reading this book.

Another reason for the unsatisfactory therapy of chronic illness is that many of these sicknesses are allergic in origin and
allergy patients commonly react adversely to chemically
derived drugs used in their treatment.

The actual number of people with allergies is far greater than
commonly realized. In any experience, allergies make up the
single largest group of unsatisfactorily treated patients today.
Some idea of the frequency with which chronic allergy exists is
indicated by the following experience. Thirty-five years ago, I
took a brief allergy history of 160 student nurses in the two
upper classes of the nursing training course. Two-thirds of these
young women, chosen in part because of their relative good
health, were shown to have had a history of some type of allergy. This survey was done in 1943, before the full range of
environmental causes of allergic reactions had become known

DR. RANDOLPH is director of the Ecologic Unit, American International Hospital, Zion, Illinois; Former Instructor in Medicine, Northwestern University
Medical School.

and before the current extent of localized and generalized allergic manifestations as well as the mental and behavioral reactions of allergic origin had been described.

The readers should know that there are two kinds of allergists today. Dr. Mandell is not the ordinary type who is principally interested in the bodily mechanisms of allergic reactions and in the drug treatment of symptoms. He is an ecologically oriented allergist, better referred to as a Clinical Ecologist, who is primarily concerned with the environmental causes of illnesses. He is an expert in how commonly eaten foods and frequently encountered environmental chemical exposures, to which millions of people are susceptible, are impairing the health and behavior of these people.

The reader should also know that we now have methods of testing that demonstrate the effects of such environmental exposures, whose impact is greatly influenced by each individual's degree of allergic susceptibility. There are various ways of approaching this type of problem. Although the simple problems can sometimes be handled on a do-it-yourself basis, professional assistance is usually preferable and often necessary. The office management of these cases, as described in this book, is usually successful in the absence of drug therapy. However, there are some extremely difficult and/or advanced cases which may require hospitalization in an ecologic unit in which all suspected and probable environmental exposures may be avoided simultaneously prior to single test reexposures that often induce an individual's typical symptoms. Avoidance of exposures to test-identified illness-causing substances is the treatment of choice.

Introduction

The field of bio-ecologic medicine as it is practiced by my colleagues and me is rapidly becoming the medicine of tomorrow. It holds great promise for those suffering from many kinds of chronic illness.

Our diagnostic techniques make it possible to identify the previously suspected causes of many forms of physical, mental, and psychosomatic disorders that heretofore have not been recognized as being the result of frequently encountered types of allergy to many substances in our environment.

This book is a message of hope for countless millions of "forgotten people" who are afflicted with diseases whose causes can be discovered and properly treated for the first time. Bio-ecologic medicine will free innumerable men, women, and children from the unwarranted burden of being labeled as psychologically inadequate or emotionally unequipped to cope with normal stress of modern living. It has been clearly demonstrated that most cases of so-called psychosomatic illness are allergic and nutritional in origin.

In their prefatory material, my distinguished colleagues Drs. Abram Hoffer and Theron G. Randolph present more of this message of hope.

—Marshall Mandell, M.D.

1
A Revolution in Medicine

Five days to allergy relief? Is that possible?

The answer is emphatically yes! In five days or less, if you follow the special diet systems and environmental control methods outlined in this book, it is quite possible that you will be able to relieve many allergies you already know you have, and discover a few new ones as well. In some specific instances, the diets and environmental control techniques may take a day or two longer, but the vast majority of people will begin to get results within five days. Moreover, you may find that many of your chronic physical, mental, and "psychosomatic" problems are allergy symptoms, and that you can now do something about them.

In a relatively simple five-day program you will be able to test yourself at home to see if allergy to foods you are eating; beverages you are drinking; molds, animal danders, pollens, dust in the air you are inhaling; and chemicals with which you are coming into contact every day are causing you serious problems with chronic fatigue that makes it difficult to get up in the morning or has you collapse, exhausted, at four o'clock in the afternoon; with depression that seems to come and go for no apparent reason; with arthritis that is bad some days and better on others; with migraine headaches that throb for hours or leave you incapacitated and unable to work for days at a time; with obesity about which it appears impossible for you to do anything; with alcoholism that drives you to drink compulsively either all day long or at specific times of the day. All these ailments, and a startling array of others, may have their origins in allergy.

Can foods, beverages, particles in the air, and chemicals really cause these types of problems? Absolutely! I have placed an extract of wheat under the tongue of a patient and promptly caused a flare-up of chronic arthritis pains; pork extract has triggered asthmatic attacks; a few drops of milk have brought on a state of deep depression. I have seen house-dust extract cause muscle pains; egg produce a stuffy, runny nose; tomato extract cause extreme mental confusion; and food coloring bring about frantic itching in some, and hyperactivity in others.

The men and women who are aware of the extent to which allergy can affect mankind are involved in a medical revolution and a brand-new field of medicine. I call it bio-ecologic medicine (biology and ecology). It combines the most exciting discoveries from the past twenty-five years in the fields of allergy, clinical ecology, nutritional therapy, preventive medicine, orthomolecular psychiatry and orthomolecular medicine, and metabology. And it outmodes many of the traditional beliefs held dear by the medical establishment for decades.

Specifically, the field of allergy has been redefined and expanded in the scope of its role in mankind's ills because foods; beverages (including water); airborne particles like dust, molds, animal danders and pollens; and the many chemicals encountered in the environment during daily activities can be the source of physical, mental, and psychological problems if a person is sensitive to any of these things.

The combined discoveries of my colleagues in various medical fields throughout the world have reached a point where it is now possible for many of our patients at last to be able to walk out and stay out of mental hospitals, get up and leave psychiatrists' couches, and discontinue the conventional treatments of highly dedicated physicians whose best efforts, when successful, have resulted only in the control or suppression of the symptoms of an illness—not the elimination of the underlying cause. Each year, with every new discovery, the importance of allergy has become increasingly appreciated by a growing number of our professional associates who form the Society for Clinical Ecology. More recently, our work has become a significant addition to the body of knowledge employed by members of the

International Academy of Preventive Medicine, the International Academy of Metabology, the Academy of Orthomolecular Psychiatry, and the Academy of Orthomolecular Medicine.

The Great Debate: Doctor vs. Doctor

There is a great (and often very heated) debate going on among the members of the medical community—a kind of old school versus new school debate. The physicians who continue to practice the conventional symptom-relieving, drug-oriented medicine they were taught in medical school (and which is still being taught in medical schools by the same team of old-guard defenders) are in conflict with the doctors who are more oriented toward discovering the cause of a problem, doing something about it, and eliminating the need for medication.

The origins of this disparity in approach and heated debate began about twenty-five years ago, when highly qualified and experienced physicians like Drs. Theron G. Randolph, Herbert Rinkel, Carleton Lee, French Hansel, Arthur Coca, and I began to realize that allergy was a much more widespread problem than anyone had ever suspected. When we began to recognize and *prove* that allergic reactions went far beyond a runny nose, hay fever, asthma, hives, or eczema and into the realm of depression, headache, chronic fatigue, compulsive eating, obesity, compulsive drinking, insomnia, hypertension, fluid retention, arthritis, duodenal ulcers, colitis, gall bladder colic, urinary tract symptoms imitating urinary infections, hyperactivity, learning disabilities, autism, retardation, multiple sclerosis, schizophrenia, and epilepsy, we triggered a tidal wave of skepticism that has not yet ebbed. Even today, after thousands of well-documented case histories have been gathered and reported in papers and at scientific meetings around the world, the vast majority of doctors persist in resisting belief in our findings.

Much like Ignatz Semmelweis' trying to convince his colleagues of the enormous importance of thoroughly washing their hands prior to assisting women in childbirth in order to eliminate fatal child-bed fever, much like Louis Pasteur's difficulties with his strange ideas about the role of invisible germs as the cause of many infectious diseases, spreading the truth about allergy as the root of much of the physical, mental, and "psychosomatic" illness that assaults our society has been an arduous uphill climb.

So if your doctor is not familiar with much of the contents of this book, do not be surprised. If he or she resists, perhaps quite strongly, the whole idea of allergy as a major factor in just about every ailment known to mankind, be forewarned. In order to recognize that allergy may play a significant role in a patient's problem, a doctor first must be aware of the scope of illnesses that allergy can encompass, and second, he must suspect allergy might be a factor in the patient's complaint.

Most doctors have not yet looked into allergy as a possible underlying cause of illness. Some of those who have looked have obstinately refused to believe what they read, and did not make the effort to learn firsthand for themselves. And unfortunately, there are others who feel quite threatened, personally and professionally, because what we have discovered is quite different from what they were taught in medical schools.

While most of the documentation about the role of allergy and environmental factors as the cause of physical, mental, and "psychosomatic" illness has been presented at scientific meetings and reported in medical journals, this book offers the public a chance to become acquainted with our discoveries firsthand and to judge for itself.

Physical, Mental, and Psychosomatic Problems

In medicine there is rarely any direct path to a major breakthrough. It took many years, and many discoveries in different fields of medicine, before some of the most important pieces of the entire picture of advanced allergic disorders and bioecologic medicine fell into place. To be sure, there were many clues that suggested the extent to which the environment (food, water, molds, dusts, pollens, and chemicals) could affect mankind: Lead poisoning was found to be responsible for retardation in children who ate paint chips off the walls, water-borne fluorides and chlorine were known to cause toxic effects, coal dust was directly linked to black lung, but the major piece of the puzzle was not discovered until some doctors stepped back and looked at the patient as a susceptible human organism interacting with his total environment—and what we saw changed the course of medicine.

Why should a person be allergic to anything that he eats, drinks, or inhales? After all, everything with which he comes into contact is derived in some form from something that is part of our Earth. The answers, we have discovered, involve mankind's increasing inability to cope with *natural* as well as *unnatural* substances in his environment.

How did this happen? For hundreds of thousands of years during the course of human evolution, changes occurred much more slowly in man's natural environment than they do in the rapidly changing chemicalized and polluted world of today. If a volcano erupted, filling the air with flames, gases, and particles and pouring forth rivers of lava, those contaminants entered the Earth's atmosphere and water, and covered some areas of land, but the Earth, still young and fresh, was able to accommodate what were, in the grand scheme of things, minor changes. The relatively limitless atmosphere, huge land masses, and enormous bodies of water easily absorbed and diluted or distributed the naturally formed volcanic pollutants. Man had sufficient time to adjust to the pollution that resulted from the activity of a natural occurrence on his planet such as a volcanic eruption. He slowly evolved over a period of hundreds of thousands of years. He adapted. He survived. When death came, it was from old age, injury, tribal war, infection, in the jaws of a saber-toothed tiger, or the cooking pot of a neighbor. When disease struck, it usually was not black lung, cancer, or coronary heart disease—these are diseases of our advanced civilization.

During the past two centuries alone, man has brought about such drastic changes in his natural environment that it has become unnatural. When organic chemistry began in the nineteenth century, a whole series of combinations of chemicals were created that were never found naturally in the environment. Pesticides, herbicides (weed killers), insecticides, waxes, preservatives, colorings, and additives, although they did the jobs they were designed for, contaminated the environment and filled man's body with residues that were totally alien to the human system. When jet fuels were developed for commercial aviation in the 1950s, combustion by-products began to be spewed across the land—by-products with no equal in the natural form. Automobiles manufactured by the millions each year compounded the problem. Oil and coal burning factories and generating plants added to this. In short, everything man eats, drinks, or inhales is now polluted with chemical agents that are foreign to his chemistry, and he is suffering the consequences of possessing a body that is incapable of handling the by-products of his amazing chemical technology.

But that is just part of the story. The second part concerns a lowered threshold of allergic resistance to physical and mental illness, and an inability to cope with the *natural* as well as the unnatural things that surround him because of an out-of-kilter body metabolism, enzyme dysfunctions, nutritional deficiencies, and hormonal imbalances.

Years ago, Weston A. Price, DDS, was involved in a nutritional study of a group of fourteen primitive societies in locations throughout the world. He uncovered an unexpected and frightening series of revelations that have extremely serious health implications for us and for future generations. One aspect of his research concerned each group's state of health *before* and *after* they began to follow some of the commonly practiced eating habits of our modern civilized society. Members of the groups of contemporary primitives he studied had perfectly formed upper and lower jaws that gave them broad dental arches, and Dr. Price rarely observed any instances of decay in their beautifully formed and properly spaced teeth. In addition, their general health and mental state was, in many respects, superior, he felt, to civilized man's.

It turned out that the basis for their superior dental health was directly related to the fact that for generations their ethnic diets had basically consisted of fresh, unprocessed, locally available foods, which included fiber-containing vegetables. However, after these same tribe members began to eat the empty (meaning vitamin- and mineral-depleted) calories of refined carbohydrates—such as granulated sugar, devitalized bleached white flour minus its germ and bran, rice without the B vitamins that are removed by polishing, canned fruits packed in syrup modified foods, and refined vegetable oils—their health picture began to alter dramatically. The most striking evidence that they were physically deteriorating was the rapid appearance of dental decay and infection in adults, and facial deformities in their offspring. Children of mothers who changed from their traditional tribal diets and adopted our modern nutrition were, for the first time in tribal history, born with abnormal facial bones: high, narrow dental arches and crowded teeth that were highly susceptible to decay and abscess formation; and for the first time in the history of the tribes, club feet and cleft palates appeared in the babies.*

The obvious questions are: What happened to the subsequent offspring of any of the women of Dr. Price's studies who went back to their natural diet? How did their next children fare?

When previously healthy mothers returned to the traditional diets of fresh, unrefined foods, the next children born to them were just as healthy as the offspring of tribe members who had not participated in the studies. They had fine, cavity-resistant teeth and good facial structure. In other words, the problems were directly related to poor maternal nutrition, and by correcting the deficiencies of the mothers' diets, the dental-facial deformities were eliminated in their next children. Thus the diet produced some form of damage to the developing fetus while it was growing within the body of a poorly nourished mother.

Simple yet brilliant nutritional studies by Dr. Price's colleague Francis Pottinger, MD, performed on three successive generations of cats to study the long-term effect of food modification in these animals were equally revelatory. Dr. Pottinger found that cats, in accordance with their carnivorous, predatory nature, *must* be nourished with raw food in order to achieve optimal health and to reproduce normally. He proved that groups of cats raised on a diet consisting of two-thirds cooked food and one-third raw food suffered from poor health and had

*Price, W. A. *Nutrition and Physical Degeneration* (Santa Monica: Price-Pottinger. Nutrition Foundation, Heritage Edition, 1971; first published 1937).

their life expectancy cut short. The third-generation cats were very much below par by the time they were only six months old. The females of the third generation were less fertile and had many miscarriages, and their offspring had much less vigor. Dr. Pottinger observed that the majority of cats raised on a diet of cooked foods suffered from many of the same ailments that afflict us: allergies, arthritis, severe fatigue, dermatitis, pyorrhea, severe dental decay, diabetes, pneumonia, nephritis, an increased rate of infection with intestinal parasites, and a marked increase in viciousness and homosexuality.*

What happened to the offspring of Dr. Pottinger's third generation of degenerating cats when they were returned from their civilized cooked diet to the natural raw diet of their healthy ancestors from many generations back? How long did it take before some of the cats or their offspring began to approach normal cat physiology and anatomy?

The cats did not respond to a sudden dietary change back to their natural foods; too many generations had elapsed from the original group of cats that comprised the first part of the nutritional experiment. The incidence of allergy had increased from 5 percent in the first generation to more than 95 percent in the third generation. It required three to four more generations of cats raised on a two-thirds raw-foods diet to reverse the damage done by three generations of poor nutrition.

Where does that leave us? We are in a precarious position at best. Man no longer has the hundreds of thousands of years his body must have to adjust gradually to changes in the environment; there have been too many changes in the quality of the air, food, and water on which he depends. Compounding matters, his diet has changed radically over the past few generations and now includes so many heat and chemically modified and nutritionally inadequate foods from poor soil that he is malnourished and in the same situation as Dr. Price's tribal members and Dr. Pottinger's cats. He is beginning to suffer

---

*Pottinger, F. M., Jr. "The effect of heat-processed foods and metabolized vitamin D milk on the dento-facial structures of experimental animals." *Am. I. Orthod. Oral Surg.* 32 (8): 467, 1946. (Reprints from Price-Pottinger Nutrition Foundation, Santa Monica, Calif.)

metabolic defects, enzymatic dysfunctions, the breakdown of disease-fighting mechanisms, and hormonal imbalances. In addition, in a weakened state, he has to deal with so many unnatural and toxic substances that his body is continually stressed. With few reserves to call on because of an inadequately nourished body, serious malfunctions often precipitate a maladapted state of hypersensitivity or allergy to many of the synthetic as well as the natural substances in his environment.

Allergens

We constantly take substances into our body from the outside world by breathing and by eating. If the air around us contains chemical vapors, fumes, or gases (as well as the molds and pollens that are normally present for long periods of time in the atmosphere), these chemical substances will enter our lungs with every breath of air we inhale. Some of the vapors or fumes invariably pass through the delicate walls of the millions upon millions of minute blood vessels (capillaries) in the lungs and enter the circulation. Once a foreign agent enters the bloodstream, all it takes is a few beats of the heart to transport it throughout the body, and expose every cell in every organ in every system of the body to it.

These foreign substances are all around us. They are made from petroleum and coal (fossil hydrocarbon fuels) from which we derive substances used for heating, cooking, insecticides, hair sprays, perfumes, waxes, polishes, detergents, room deodorizers, gasoline, paint thinner, tar, plastics, lubricants, asphalt, cement, and adhesives; and in cigarette smoke, which pollutes the air in the home with hundreds of toxic materials from the combustion of chemically treated tobacco and cigarette paper.

The mouth, the portal of entry for the gastrointestinal tract, is the starting point for a passageway about twenty-five to thirty feet long that ends with the anus, the muscles of which control the emptying of the lower bowel. During the entire digestive process, there is constant activity on the part of the body to break down and absorb proteins, carbohydrates, and fat nutrients, as well as the vitamins and minerals to sustain itself. Complex proteins are converted into simple amino acids and complex starches are converted into simple sugars that are ultimately absorbed by passing through the walls of the capillary blood vessels in the lining of the bowel. During this process, other materials that we ingest, such as artificial coloring and flavoring agents, drugs, food preservatives, and insecticides to which we may be allergic or chemically susceptible, also get absorbed through the delicate blood vessels in the walls of the intestines. Once something is absorbed into the bloodstream from the digestive tract, it travels in the blood through the liver and to the heart, and then is transported within minutes to all parts of the body including the brain, which has a very rich blood supply and, therefore, a heavy exposure to substances that have entered the bloodstream.

Finding the Problem

The causes of many physical, mental, and "psychosomatic" disorders can often be uncovered by performing a series of relatively simple *symptom-duplicating* tests, which can clearly demonstrate the cause-and-effect relationships between an exposure to a food, beverage (including tap water), particles or chemicals in the air and your reactions to them.

During cause-and-effect testing, my colleagues and I have produced arthritis, visual blurring, dizziness, hyperactivity, and abdominal pain from exposure to beef and food coloring; epilepsy symptoms have been evoked in the hospital following the ingestion of wheat and other foods. Various symptoms of schizophrenia, including the catatonic state, have been produced from exposure to common foods and molds and to fumes of chemicals often used in household and building maintenance products; migraine headache symptoms with fatigue and depression from coffee, onions, and many other foods, in addition to the chlorine present in drinking water and in household bleaching agents; weakness, fatigue, and confusion from brewer's yeast and foods from which alcoholic beverages are manufactured; rectal-genital itching and burning from exposure to orange, pork, tomatoes, and milk. I have induced ex-

treme irritability, restlessness, and uncontrolled violent outbursts of anger associated with physical violence from egg and
soy. Asthma has resulted from tests with foods including
"bland" and "innocent" ones that are often part of what is
thought to be a hypoallergenic diet—for instance, potato, rice,
lettuce, squash, and lamb.

Nasal inhalation ("sniff") tests with pollens, molds, animal
danders, and house dust have caused immediate eye, ear, nose,
throat, and sinus symptoms and episodes of "out-of-season" hay
fever and asthma, along with completely unexpected nervous
and mental symptoms, which have continued to fascinate me
ever since I first observed these very important central nervous
system reactions to common airborne allergens.

A healthy individual reacts to foods, beverages, and the pollens and molds in the air, environmental chemicals, etc., by a
complex and incompletely understood process of adaptation
that somehow permits the body to function without any apparently harmful reactions to these insults. But the body that is
predisposed by heredity and has been poorly nourished can
meet stresses of this nature head on for only a limited period of
time, which varies greatly from person to person. When stress
almost never lets up, when the offending foods, beverages,
water and air contaminants are continuously present, such a
person breaks down on a biochemical level and may have problems all over his body. Eventually, he makes his way to the
doctor's office, usually complaining of a combination of symptoms. He may have been adapting for years and now he has
come to a stage in the evolution of his health problem that he
and his physician incorrectly identify as "the onset" of his illness.

It is not unusual for a woman to enter a doctor's office and say,
"I feel tired and tense. I get headaches, dizziness, and visual
blurring. My face gets puffy and my head and nose get blocked
up. My ears hurt and I hear ringing sounds in them on and off.
I get stomach cramps, bloating, nausea, and belching with a
repeat taste of some foods. I am gassy. I am very uncomfortable
with rectal and vaginal itching. My left ankle and right knee
hurt, and my hands often become quite stiff."

Faced with such a bizarre assortment of apparently unrelated symptoms, most physicians would probably throw their hands up and assume that this woman was a proper candidate for their list of patients with widespread psychosomatic disorders or severe neurotic problems, with an inability to cope with life's normal stresses. Some patients are regarded as multiple-complaint hypochondriacs, and other physicians have less pleasant and most unscientific descriptions for patients having these combinations of symptoms. In my experience, I have found that these patients have very real disorders and genuine illnesses of the kind that have been inaccurately diagnosed and inappropriately treated in thousands of medical offices, clinics, emergency rooms, and hospitals every day of the year. Even though our standard medical textbooks do not yet describe ailments consisting of such apparently unrelated symptoms that cause so much human misery and loss of valuable living time, they do occur in millions of people who do not have to remain ill and who do not have to endlessly take symptom-relieving medications and who do not have to spend countless wasted hours with clinical psychologists and psychiatrists. I know these puzzling and seemingly bizarre combinations of symptoms are real! I have diagnosed and treated thousands of them. In testing in my laboratory under controlled conditions, in the hospital, and in the patients' homes, the symptoms of these complex problems have been made to flare up as a direct result of a specific test exposure to a dietary substance or to some commonly encountered environmental chemical material. My colleagues, my students, and I have reproduced these symptoms by testing for allergy to foods, beverages, airborne particles, and environmental chemical agents.

Some people come to the Alan Mandell Center for Bio-Ecologic Diseases hoping that something can be done for them or for a loved one in a situation where sheer desperation has led them to try "anything," including me, as the last-resort in their search for better health. Other people come to the Center knowing that their problems are somehow related to the food they are eating, beverages they are drinking, inhalants they are breathing, or chemical substances to which they are exposed.

There are highly observant patients who are quick to tell me that they get dizzy, tense, and nauseous when they are caught in traffic jams in which the combustion products of gasoline and diesel fumes are permeating the air. Some of the people who are sensitive to chemicals are fully aware of the fact that they cannot stand to be in a freshly painted room or in a room where hair spray has just been applied or in the presence of a person who has recently applied a perfumed cosmetic or spray. Often they are extremely uncomfortable in vague ways that they cannot quite describe when they are exposed to floor and furniture polish, air fresheners, marking pens, insect sprays, moth flakes, disinfectants, chlorine bleach, and oven cleaners. I see patients who know that entering a moldy basement will cause them to develop a tight chest, itching eyes, a sore throat, a runny nose, and blocked-up ears. Others are aware of the fact that tobacco smoke gives them nausea and headaches, may make them irritable and tired, and often produces visual blurring.

The major problem with most chemically susceptible patients who have made such important observations is that they do not have a comprehensive overview of the many factors involved. They do not know what can and should be done about their problem. They do not know that if gasoline fumes can cause nausea and other symptoms, that many other petroleum-derived substances, including the fumes emitted by their home-heating furnace or kitchen range, both using natural gas, can also cause many difficulties which may or may not include the nausea caused by gasoline. Patients know that specific locations in their house seem to be related to the appearance of physical and mental symptoms, but they have not made the connection between the presence of many types of airborne molds in their immediate environment and the appearance of symptoms. It has never occurred to them that breathing in the molds (mildew) to which they are allergic can lead to bodywide manifestations after the mold particles (which collect on the sticky mucus in the back of the throat) have been swallowed, digested, and absorbed into their system through the membranes of the intestinal tract.

Table 1 lists the most common symptoms that have been reproduced by various types of testing for allergies at the Alan Mandell Center for Bio-Ecologic Diseases. Table 2 lists many of the symptoms and syndromes that have been experienced by allergic men, women, and children after exposure to foods, beverages, inhalants, and a variety of chemicals. If these symptoms seem to encompass just about every ailment and complaint known to man, that is because bio-ecologic illness often is at the root of just about all types of human malfunctioning.

More than 2,000 years ago, Hippocrates, the father of medicine, wrote: ". . . it appears to me necessary to every physician to be skilled in nature, and to strive to know, if he would wish to perform his duties, what man is in relation to the articles of food and drink, and to his other occupations, and what are the effects of each of them to everyone."*

Table 1: Symptoms Reproduced in Patients by Testing for Allergies

1. *Skin:* Itching, burning, flushing, hot flashes, warmth, coldness, tingling, sweating behind neck, hives, blisters, blotches, red spots, pimples.
2. *Ear, nose, throat:* Nasal obstruction, sneezing, nasal itching, runny nose, postnasal drip, sore or dry or tickling throat, clearing throat, itching palate, hoarseness, hacking cough, fullness or ringing or popping of ears, itching deep within ears, earache with red or normal eardrums, intermittent deafness, loss of some tones, sounds much louder, fluid accumulation in the middle ear, dizziness, vertigo, imbalance.
3. *Eye:* Blurring of vision, temporary loss of vision, double vision, spots before the eyes, pain in or behind the eyes, watery eyes, excessive tear secretion, crossing of eyes, glare hurts eyes, colors look brighter; eyelids twitching, itching, drooping, or swollen; redness and swelling of the lids.
4. *Respiratory:* Shortness of breath, tightness in the chest, not enough air getting into the lungs, wheezing cough, mucus formation in bronchial tubes, rattling sounds or vibrations in the chest.
5. *Cardiovascular:* Pounding heart, increased heart rate, skipped beats, flushing, hot flashes, pallor; warmth, coldness, tingling, redness or blueness of hands; faintness; pain in front of the heart; pain in the left arm, shoulder, neck, and jaw traveling down to the wrist (pseudo-heart attack pain).
6. *Gastrointestinal:* Dryness of mouth, hunger, thirst, increased sali-

*McCarrison, R. *Nutrition and Health* (London: Faber, 1964).

vation, canker sores, metallic taste in mouth, stinging tongue, toothache, burping, retasting foods, ulcer symptoms, heartburn, indigestion, infantile colic, nausea, vomiting, difficulty in swallowing, rumbling in abdomen, constipation, abdominal pain, spastic colitis, "emotional" colitis, gall bladder colic, cramps, diarrhea, passing gas, mucus or blood through the rectum, itching or burning of rectum or anus.

7. *Genitourinary:* Frequent, urgent, or painful urination; inability to control bladder; bedwetting; vaginal discharge; itching, swelling, redness or pain in the genitals; painful intercourse.

8. *Musculoskeletal:* Fatigue, generalized muscular weakness, muscle pain, joint pain, joint swelling with local redness, stiffness, joint deformity, arthritis soreness, chest pain, backache, neck muscle spasm, shoulder muscle spasm, generalized spasticity, limping gait, limitation of motion.

9. *Nervous System:* Headache, migraine, compulsively sleepy, drowsy, groggy, confused, dizzy, loss of balance, staggering gait, slow, sluggish, dull, unable to concentrate, depressed, crying; tense, angry, irritable, anxious, panic, stimulated, aggressive, overactive, frightened, restless, manic, hyperactive with learning disability, jittery, convulsions, head feels full or enlarged, floating sensation, silliness, poor memory, variations in reading ability, reading without comprehension, misreading, variations in penmanship legibility, feeling of separateness or apartness from others, amnesia for words or numbers or names, hallucinations, delusions, paranoid state, stammering or stuttering speech, claustrophobia, paralysis, catatonic state, perceptual dysfunctions, typical symptoms of mental retardation.

Table 2: Typical Allergic Symptoms*

A. Headache
   1. Migraine
   2. Vascular

*The symptoms in Table 2 may also be due to a variety of other causes, but allergy and addiction, as well as metabolic-nutritional disorders, are major causes that most certainly must be ruled out. Doing so can save time and considerable sums of money that would be spent on a series of expensive and possibly dangerous and uncomfortable diagnostic procedures in offices, laboratories, or hospitals.

      3. Histamine
      4. Tension
      5. "Emotional"
      6. Muscle spasm

B. Ophthalmic
      1. Eye pain
      2. Photophobia
      3. Episodic blurring of vision
      4. Transitory refractive changes
      5. Tearing

C. Otologic
      1. Serous otitis
      2. Tinnitus
      3. Menière's syndrome
      4. Hearing loss
      5. Vertigo

D. Respiratory
      1. Laryngeal edema
      2. Asthma
      3. Postnasal discharge
      4. Allergic tracheitis
      5. Allergic laryngitis
      6. Allergic rhinitis

E. Cardiovascular
      1. Extrasystoles
      2. Tachycardia
      3. Palpitation
      4. Episodic syncope
      5. Generalized angio-edema
      6. Angio-edema of lungs, liver, etc.
      7. Flushing, chilling

F. Gastrointestinal
      1. Cheilitis
      2. Aphthous stomatitis
      3. Aerophagia
      4. Nausea
      5. Vomiting
      6. Heartburn
      7. Indigestion
      8. Gassiness

    9. Abdominal pain
  10. Cramps
  11. Diarrhea
  12. Pruritus ani
  13. Irritable bowel
  14. Spastic colon
  15. Mucous colitis
  16. Nervous stomach
  17. Food intolerances

G. Dermatologic
    1. Urticaria
    2. Atopic dermatitis
    3. Neurodermatitis
    4. Adult acne
    5. Erythema multiforme
    6. Skin lesions of porphyria
    7. Hand dermatitis
    8. Nondescript syndromes

H. Muscular
    1. Muscle spasm
    2. Muscle pain
    3. Muscle cramps
    4. Muscle weakness
    5. Nuchal pain or rigidity
    6. Undue fatigue
    7. Sluggishness

I. Cerebral depression
    1. Acute and chronic depression
    2. Drowsiness approaching narcolepsy
    3. Episodic dullness or dreaminess
    4. Learning disorders
    5. Tension-fatigue syndrome
    6. Minimal brain dysfunction

J. Cerebral stimulation
    1. Restlessness
    2. Nervousness
    3. Jitteriness
    4. Insomnia
    5. Hyperactivity
    6. Behavior problems

K. Psychiatric
    1. Feelings of apartness
    2. Floating sensation
    3. Episodic amnesia
    4. Pathologically poor memory
    5. Inability to concentrate
    6. Personality changes
L. Urological
    1. Frequency
    2. Dysuria
    3. Nocturia
    4. Enuresis
M. Hematological
    1. Anemia
    2. Neutropenia
    3. Purpura

Are You Allergic?—A Questionnaire*

This is a five-part questionnaire designed to help you find out whether you may be allergic, and if so, on an investigatory basis, to see if you can't get some clues as to what your allergies may be.

PART I GENERAL HISTORY

To the best of your recollection, when you were a child:

	Yes	No
•Did you wet the bed?		
•Did you have eczema or any other chronic skin trouble?		
•Did you have colic?		
•Were you a feeding problem?		
•Did you have frequent ear aches?		

*Adapted from "Chronic Urticaria" by Alfred V. Zamm, published in *Clinical Ecology*. (Also published in *Cutis* magazine, 1/72, 2/72, and 5/73.) Reprinted by permission of author and publisher.

•Did you have croup?
•Did you have bronchitis or chest colds?
•Did you have persistent coughs?
•Did you have hay fever?
•Did you have frequent attacks of "sto-
    machache," diarrhea, or vomiting?
•Did you have circles under the eyes?
•Did you have learning disabilities?

If you answered "yes" to any of the above questions, there is a good chance that you were showing signs and symptoms of childhood allergy.

Do you notice that your trouble begins or is aggravated:

	Yes	No
•During prolonged periods of damp weather?		
•When you are near hay or straw (as at the circus, in a barn, near a hay stack, on a hay ride)? When you go into an old, damp, musty house, a damp basement, a shed or cellar? When you enter a closet in which are stored old shoes, unused luggage, gloves, or other leather goods? If you eat cheese, mush-rooms, cantaloupe, vinegar, or sauer-kraut or drink buttermilk or other fer-mented beverages (beer, wine, whiskey)? When you sit in old over-stuffed furniture?		
•When you are near dry leaves or compost?		
•Are you better when the snow is on the ground?		

If you answered "yes" to any of the above questions, chances are you have an allergy to molds.

Do you notice that your trouble begins or is aggravated:

	Yes	No
•When the house is being cleaned or swept?		
•When rugs are being beaten?		
•When the bed is being made or the mattress turned?		
•During spring house cleaning?		
•When the first cold snap of autumn comes and heat is turned on?		
•In such places as theaters, churches, grocery stores, department stores, libraries, or your bedroom where dust is noted?		

If you answered "yes" to any of the above questions, chances are you have an allergy to house dust.

Do you notice that your trouble begins or is aggravated:

	Yes	No
•When lying on a feather pillow?		
•When fluffing pillows?		
•When using a down comforter?		
•When you are near chickens, ducks, geese, pigeons, parrots, turkeys, canaries, or other birds?		
•When you are around anyone who works with poultry or other fowl?		

If you answered "yes" to any of the above questions, chances are you have an allergy to feathers.

Do you notice that your trouble begins or is aggravated:

	Yes	No
•When you are around any of the following animals: dogs, cats, horses, goats, rabbits, cows, hogs, sheep?		
•When you handle or come into contact with any of the following: furs, rugs,		

certain articles of clothing, dress
goods, blankets, gloves, hats, toy animals, or brushes?

If you answered "yes" to any of the above questions, chances
are you are allergic to animal hairs, danders and odors.

Do you notice that your trouble begins or is aggravated:

	Yes	No
•When using face, talcum, body, bath, or tooth powder?		
•In beauty salons or barber shops?		
•When you are around people who use a lot of powder or perfume?		

If you answered "yes" to any of the above questions, chances
are you are allergic to petroleum-derived chemicals or to orris
root, which is the base of some of these products.

Do you notice that your trouble begins or is aggravated:

	Yes	No
•When you handle or are around animal or poultry feed?		
•When you use certain hair wave sets, shampoos, or tonics?		

If you answered "yes" to any of the above questions, you may
be allergic to cottonseed and/or flaxseed.

Do you notice that your trouble begins or is aggravated:

	Yes	No
•When you smoke?		
•When you are around those who are smoking?		
•When in nightclubs or other smoky places?		

If you answered "yes" to any of the above, chances are you are
allergic to tobacco, or susceptible to the chemicals employed in

22

growing tobacco or manufacturing cigarettes, or the chemicals in the paper in which the tobacco is wrapped.

Do you notice that your trouble begins or is aggravated:

	Yes	No
•When you are exposed to household insect powder or sprays?		
•When you are exposed to powders, sprays, or crystals used for mothproofing purposes?		
•When you are exposed to dusting powders, sprays used in the garden or on crops?		

If you answered "yes" to any of the above questions, chances are you are allergic to pyrethrum, derris root, paradichlorobenzene or highly toxic insect sprays.

PART II GASTROINTESTINAL SYSTEM

	Yes	No
•Do you frequently belch after meals?		
•Do you often have indigestion and bloating following meals?		
•Is there any food that you feel disagrees with you each time you eat it?		
•Do you often have attacks of diarrhea?		
•Do you often have constipation or chronic constipation?		
•Do you suffer with cramping pains in your lower abdomen?		
•Have you ever been told you have mucous colitis?		
•Have you ever been told you have gall bladder disease?		
•Have you ever had acute pain in the abdomen associated with hives and itching of the skin?		

•Do you suspect any food of causing or ag-
gravating your condition?

•Are there any foods that you dislike?

•Are there any foods you crave, love or overindulge in or eat frequently because
you like them so much?

•Is there any seasonal food (for example,
strawberries) that you overindulge in?

•Are there any foods you find difficult to
digest?

•Do any foods you eat cause nausea, vomiting, diarrhea, heartburn, belching, gas,
cramps, hives, skin rashes, headache?

•Are you on any type of special diet at present?

•Are you uncomfortable if you do not eat on
time?

•Do you feel good after you eat?

•Do you feel better if you skip a meal or
fast?

•Do alcoholic beverages make you ill?

•Do alcoholic beverages take symptoms
away?

•Do you get hangover symptoms from a single drink?

If you answered "yes" to any of the above questions, chances
are you suffer from food allergy.

PART III FOCAL INFECTION HISTORY

	Yes	No

•Are you conscious of a foul odor in your
nose?

•Do you have a dripping from the back of
your nose into your throat which has a
"sickening sweet" taste or is yellow or
green?

- •Have you ever been treated for "sinus trouble"?
- •Do you have any bad teeth?
- •Do you have bad breath at times?
- •Do your gums bleed?
- •Do you have bad tonsils?
- •Do your ears drain?
- •Have you been told that you have gall bladder trouble?
- •Do you have increased frequency of urination?
- •Does urinating cause a burning sensation?
- •As far as you know, do you have pus in your urine?
- •Are you bothered with a genital discharge?
- •As far as you know, do you have an infection in any part of your body?

(For Women Only)

- •Have you been told that you have a laceration or erosion of your womb or that you need to be cauterized?

(For Men Only)

- •Have you ever been told that you have an infection of your prostate gland?
- •Do you have low back pain?
- •Do you have pains, at times, in your testicles?
- •Do you have pains, at times, at the tip of your penis?
- •Do you have trouble starting stream when urinating?

If you answered "yes" to any of the above, chances are you suffer from an allergy that manifests itself in physical ailments.

PART IV PETROLEUM PRODUCTS*

Coal, Oil, Gas, and Combustion Products

	Love or crave	Dislike or hate	Made sick by	Feel good from	Feel neutral about
Massive outdoor exposures to coal smoke					
Smoke in steam railroad stations, train sheds, and yards					
Smoke from coal-burning stoves, furnaces, or fireplaces					
Odors of natural gas fields					
Odors of escaping utility gas					
Odors of burning utility gas					
Odors of gasoline					
Garage fumes and odors					
Automotive or motor boat exhausts					
Odor of naphtha, cleaning fluids, or lighter fluids					
Odor of recently cleaned clothing, upholstery, or rugs					

*(The first extensive questionnaire of this type was prepared by my dear friend and mentor Theron G. Randolph, M.D., who coined the term "chemical susceptibility" and conducted basic and advanced studies in this extremely important field, which has grown from his basic concepts. Most of this data appears in the current edition of *Clinical Ecology*, L. Dickey, ed. [Springfield, Ill.: Charles C. Thomas, 1976].)

Odor of naphtha-containing soaps					
Odor of nail polish or nail polish remover					
Odor of brass, metal, or shoe polish					
Odor of fresh newspapers					
Odor of kerosene					
Odor of kerosene or fuel-oil lamps or stoves					
Odor of kerosene or fuel-oil space heaters or furnaces					
Diesel engine fumes from trains, buses, trucks, or boats					
Lubricating greases or crude oil					
Fumes from automobiles burning an excessive amount of oil					
Fumes from burning greasy rags					
Odors of smudge pots as road markers or frost inhibitors					

Mineral Oil, Petroleum Jelly, Waxes, and Combustion Products

	Love or crave	Dislike or hate	Made sick by	Feel good from	Feel neutral about
Mineral oil as contained in hand lotions and medications					
Mineral oil as a laxative					
Cold cream or face or foundation cream					

	Love or crave	Dislike or hate	Made sick by	Feel good from	Feel neutral about
Petroleum jelly or petrolatum-containing ointments					
Odors of floor, furniture, or bowling alley wax					
Odors of glass wax or similar glass cleaners					
Fumes from burning wax candles					
Odors from dry garbage incinerators					

Asphalts, Tars, Resins, and Dyes

	Love or crave	Dislike or hate	Made sick by	Feel good from	Feel neutral about
Fumes from tarred roofs and roads					
Asphalt pavements in hot weather					
Tar-containing soaps, shampoos, and ointments					
Odors of inks, carbon paper, typewriter ribbons, and stencils					
Dyes in clothing and shoes					
Dyes in cosmetics (lipstick, mascara, rouge, powder, other)					

Disinfectants, Deodorants, and Detergents

	Love or crave	Dislike or hate	Made sick by	Feel good from	Feel neutral about
Odor of public or household disinfectants and deodorants					

Odor of phenol (carbolic acid) or Lysol					
Phenol-containing lotions or ointments					
Injectable materials containing phenol as a preservative					
Fumes from burning creosote-treated wood (railroad ties)					
Household detergents					

Miscellaneous

	Love or crave	Dislike or hate	Made sick by	Feel good from	Feel neutral about
Air conditioning					
Ammonia fumes					
Odor of moth balls					
Odor of insect repellant candles					
Odor of termite extermination treatment					
Odor of DDT-containing insecticide sprays					
Odor of chlordane, lindane, parathion, dieldrin, or other insecticide sprays					
Odor of the fruit and vegetable sections of supermarkets					
Odor of chlorinated water					
Drinking of chlorinated water					

Fumes of chlorine gas					
Odor of Clorox and other hypochlorite bleaches					
Fumes from sulfur-processing plants					
Fumes of sulfur dioxide					

Pine

	Love or crave	Dislike or hate	Made sick by	Feel good from	Feel neutral about
Odor of Christmas trees and other indoor evergreen decorations					
Odor of knotty pine interiors					
Odor from sanding or working with pine or cedar wood					
Odor of cedar-scented furniture polish					
Odor of pine-scented household deodorants					
Odor of pine-scented bath oils, shampoos, or soaps					
Odor of turpentine or turpentine-containing paints					
Fumes from burning pine cones or wood					

If you checked any column except the "feel neutral" column, you are probably allergic/susceptible to chemicals of various types.

PART V FOOD-DERIVED ALCOHOLIC BEVERAGES

	Yes	No
•Do you drink an alcoholic beverage at least once a day?		
•Do you find you crave an alcoholic beverage?		
•Do you always drink the same type of alcoholic beverage every time you drink?		
•Does any drink make your ill or cause any kind of symptom?		
•Did any alcoholic beverage make you ill when you were first learning to drink?		
•Do complaints appear a short time after you drink?		
•Do symptoms appear many hours later?		
•Do symptoms appear the following morning?		
•Does alcoholic beverage at any time seem to take away any physical or mental discomfort that you may have?		
•Does even a small amount of alcohol have an effect on you?		
•Are you an alcoholic?		

If you answered "yes" to any of the above questions, you may be allergic to any or all of the foods in the alcoholic beverage. If alcohol in small amounts has any special effects on you, it is quite possible that you have some health problem, physical or mental, caused by the foods or the brewer's yeast from which the beverages were made.

2
New Discoveries in Allergy

About twenty-five years ago a group of trailblazing, ecologically-oriented physicians began developing new concepts, confirming each other's observations, and determining new methods of treatment that would be effective for patients suffering from allergies. I know personally most of the physicians engaged in bio-ecologic medicine and have had the privilege of sharing and working out many ideas with these distinguished physicians. Unfortunately, space does not permit me to include all of the contributors, or to present their contributions in their entirety but I have included some of the most exciting and less medically technical material that I felt would be of particular interest to the nonmedical community.

Again, I wish to state that if your personal physician is not acquainted with these discoveries, don't be surprised. Our work is unique and at first introduction appears to be so revolutionary in concept that your physician may not have a very clear picture of it, or he or she may be completely uninformed on this subject because the more conventional medical orientation does not yet include our contributions in the field of human health.

Scratch Tests Are Inaccurate

Did you know that there is general agreement among all allergists that the traditional methods of skin testing are very unreliable in the diagnosis of food allergy? In fact, many allergists are reluctant to do any food testing at all because this procedure is, at best, only twenty percent accurate. To state it another way, conventional skin tests for determining specific food allergies give results that are wrong more than 80 percent of the time.

The late Dr. Arthur Coca, a distinguished immunologist of world renown with many years of professional practice and research in the fields of bio-ecologic illness, immunology and allergy, discovered the reason why scratch, prick-puncture, and intradermal methods are so unreliable in the diagnosis of food allergy. Dr. Coca found that not everyone has substances in their blood known as *reagins.* Reagins are a kind of allergic antibody which may be formed in response to exposure to various foods for which a person may be tested. Reagins may react with the test material, which is introduced into the outer layer of the skin producing visible skin reactions (a localized red area on the skin, or a mosquito-bite-like bump) that are widely believed to identify substances to which an individual is allergic. Dr. Coca found, however, that many people with food allergies did not react to skin tests for many of the foods to which they were allergic. Why? Because if a person who was allergic to, say, pork showed no visible reaction to a skin test performed with pork extract, this *false-negative* test signified that anti-pork reagins were not present in the body at the time the test was performed, despite the fact that the individual had definite allergic symptoms after eating pork. On the other hand, another patient might be tested with pork extract and develop a definite reaction called a *false-positive* at the point where the extract was introduced into the outer layer of the skin, and yet not react to pork at all.

All very confusing. So confusing, in fact, that a typical patient may enter an allergist's office and actually receive a brief pretest lecture on the inadequacies of the testing about to take place. The doctor may indicate that a series of skin tests are to be performed on the patient, but that, in the case of food allergy, they really cannot be relied upon. After the patient undergoes a series of tests, the results are evaluated, and in the case of foods that gave no reaction, the allergist may inquire whether or not the test-negative foods ever bother the patient and base some recommendations on the patient's observations. But on the test-positive results, the doctor has to ask similar questions. All very hit-and-miss, with the 20 percent accuracy figure being more luck than anything else. Ultimately, the traditional allergist has to rely on the patient's observations based on his or her experience with various foods.

Bio-ecologic allergists no longer use the old scratch, prick-puncture, and intradermal methods. We don't have to. We can now test with great accuracy by using a different method of testing that totally outmodes traditional testing and the need for guesswork on the part of physician and patient.

Cyclic, Addictive, and Fixed Allergies

The late Dr. Herbert Rinkel solved some of the biggest mysteries in the field of bio-ecologic illness and allergy. He was a highly trained and exceptionally well-disciplined observer whose brilliant insights and tireless investigation have left physicians and patients alike a priceless heritage.

Dr. Rinkel found there are several types of allergies. Some allergies depend on the amount of exposure to a food, beverage, inhalant, or chemical: If you have an allergy to, say, corn and you eat corn in some form once a week, you may not have any reaction to it. But if you eat corn flakes for breakfast, corn bread for lunch, and corn on the cob at dinner, with cornstarch or corn sugar (glucose/dextrose) in the dessert, you may build up to a whopping corn reaction. This is why some patients will come to me and say, "Bread bothers me, but not all the time. If I eat it for four or five days, I get into trouble. If I stop eating it, I am all right again, and I can eat it again." What these patients are really saying is that they build up to a specific level after four or five days and have cumulative symptoms; if they then discontinue eating bread, the overload of the wheat or yeast allergen drops down very quickly so that they can tolerate it again in this *cyclic* kind of eating pattern.

On the other hand, you may have a type of allergy in which you eat the same foods quite frequently and have developed an allergic type of addiction (an *addictive* allergy). Most people with food addiction are completely unaware that this process is taking place in their body. If an addicted person misses a meal that would normally include the food to which he is allergic, *allergic-addictive* withdrawal symptoms appear. In order not to experience the discomfort of a withdrawal reaction, a person actually has to keep eating the food to which he is allergic in order to stave off withdrawal symptoms. Dr. Rinkel described this blocking phenomenon, where the appearance of symptoms is prevented by repeated exposures to an offending substance, as *masking*. The person suffering from a severe degree of the addictive type of allergy is aware of his addicted state. He may refer to himself as a "foodaholic" or "junk-food junkie."

The third type of allergy is one in which you have a *fixed* reaction to a food. That is, every time you eat it, you react. It does not matter whether you have eaten the food along with another food, or whether you have only a small amount, you react.

Dr. Rinkel also discovered an aspect of allergy that had puzzled physicians for years. He found that most people who give up by choice or happen not to come into contact with a food to which they are allergic for a period of four to five days develop a period of acute *hypersensitivity,* and if they don't wait long enough for this acutely hypersensitive state to wear off (usually a few weeks), on reexposure they may have a tremendous allergic reaction during which their symptoms may flare up explosively—much worse than ever before. Their chronic low-grade or moderate symptoms usually are converted to severe or acute symptoms if offending foods are avoided for four to five days.

Dr. Rinkel developed an ingenious method of diet therapy for food allergy which he named the Rotary Diversified Diet. His diet technique (and I use it throughout this book) consists of eating only one single food at a time at each meal, and waiting at least four days between exposures to that same food. Not only does separating exposures to the same food for at least four days put you in a hypersensitive state with regard to that food so that you will know right away when you eat it, if you are allergic to it, but conversely, it allows you to find out if you are *not* highly allergic to a food if you don't react when you do eat it. In addition, because we now know that people who suffer from allergies are prone to getting new ones if they overload their system with repeated exposures to the same thing, Dr. Rinkel's Rotary Diversified Diet automatically helps prevent new allergies by keeping at least four days between exposures.*

A New Method of Testing and Treatment

Dr. Coca's discovery that not everybody has the reagins to react positively to skin tests when an allergy is present made new methods of testing necessary. Drs. Lawrence D. Dickey and Guy O. Pfeiffer tried testing patients for allergies by placing a tiny drop of extract of various foods, beverages, dusts, molds, pollens, and chemicals, to which they might be allergic, under their tongue.** And it worked! With one to four drops of, say, grape extract or chocolate extract placed under the tongue, the patient who is allergic to the test material begins to develop symptoms usually within a few minutes. In almost every instance, the patient cannot taste or smell anything that would indicate what the test material is. What is most exciting is that the allergic reactions to the test usually duplicate the type of reaction the patient would have experienced immediately or hours later if he had come into contact with the food, beverage, dust, mold, pollen, or chemical on his own! There are no red welts or redness of the skin to indicate there is an allergy (the old traditional, inaccurate skin test); instead, there often is an immediate, dramatic response in the form of actual symptoms familiar to the patient, such as coughing, sneezing, depression, headache, weakness, fatigue, joint pain, abdominal discomfort, etc.

*I prefer a five- to seven-day interval whenever possible because many patients do better with this spacing between foods.
**Drs. Dickey and Pfeiffer modified the Rinkel/Lee skin test injection technique. The use of the sublingual route in treatment was pioneered by Dr. French Hansel.

How to Stop an Allergic Reaction Without Medication

Dr. Carleton Lee of St. Joseph, Missouri, a giant among the pioneer researchers in the field of bio-ecologic medicine and allergy,* developed the *neutralizing dose* technique of blocking or reversing allergic symptoms throughout the body.

At the time of his research, Dr. Lee was investigating cases of known and probable food allergy by giving each patient a group of skin tests of different strengths of the same extract to see if any particular dose of test material could be diagnostically useful. For example, he would inject into the outer layer of the skin five to ten or more doses of differing strengths of either wheat, milk, egg, orange, beef, coffee, or potato extract. He would use solutions that were diluted from 1:100, 1:500, 1:2500 all the way up to 1:8 million, 1:40 million, 1:200 million, and higher. During the course of his testing, Dr. Lee found that a number of the patients being tested mentioned that some or all of their usual symptoms, which were present when they came into the office, had become much milder or had completely disappeared during their testing. Other patients who received a set of various strengths of solutions prepared from the same food reacted to these tests with familiar symptoms that had not been present before the tests were given. And there were some individuals whose already present symptoms became much worse.

With clinical thoroughness, Dr. Lee repeated and then extended his studies. He quickly learned that it was possible to provoke and relieve many types of reactions, and the relieving doses could be used as a form of treatment in some cases. (Dr. Lee's discoveries helped to outmode the inaccurate traditional skin tests and replace them with a highly accurate alternative. His contribution in this area of allergy treatment completely revolutionizes some aspects of conventional treatment.) He found, for example, that if a patient was experiencing an aller-

*Dr. Lee was given the Society for Clinical Ecology's highest award—the Jonathan Forman award for distinguished service to humanity.

gic coughing spasm caused by pharyngeal (throat) or bronchial sensitivity to wheat, he could give this patient an injection consisting of a small dose (one to four drops) of highly diluted wheat extract and thereby often eliminate the cough. The wheat extract blocked or reversed the allergic coughing in the patient's respiratory tract and the patient often felt better almost immediately! Again, why this works remains a medical mystery, but it does.

Actually, I have found that many of my patients neutralize their own symptoms unknowingly. For example, one of my patients, J.G., forty-eight years old, was reluctant to discuss what he believed to be an important but rather peculiar observation that he had made, because he felt that he might be embarrassed by my possible response. He was convinced, he told me, that a very small piece of bread, less than one square inch of a regular slice, which he always ate at 2:00 AM, usually cleared his regularly appearing early morning attacks of asthma, which invariably woke him up at this time. Being fully acquainted with Dr. Lee's discovery of the neutralizing phenomenon and having employed it frequently myself, I concluded that my patient was doing his own at-home asthma-relieving neutralization, which he had discovered completely on his own: He had an *addictive* craving for wheat at 2:00 AM and a small amount of wheat blocked his wheat withdrawal symptom—an acute attack of allergic bronchial asthma.

On the following page are drawings of a tree and of the alphabet done by an above-average ten-year-old child who was very sensitive to some substance(s) in chemically derived petroleum alcohol (ethanol). I tested her for ethanol (ethyl alcohol) allergy by injecting one drop of this petroleum alcohol into the outer layer of her skin.* This constitutes a fairly accurate screening test for the presence of chemical susceptibility; the test was developed by Dr. Theron G. Randolph. Drawings I and II represent her allergic reactions. Drawings III and IV repre-

*Presented to the Symposium on Alcohol of the Seventh Inter-American Conference on Toxicology and Occupational Medicine, Miami, August 18, 1970, and published in the *Journal of the International Academy of Metabology,* 2:1, March 1973.

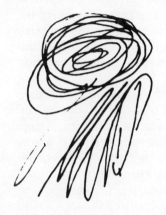

Drawing I   Provocation
Ethanol .05cc 1:250

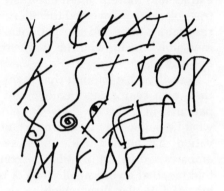

Drawing II   Provocation

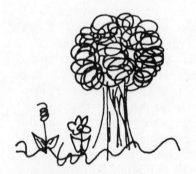

Drawing III   Neutralization
Ethanol .05cc 1:30,000

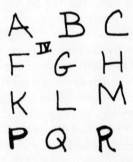

Drawing IV   Neutralization

sent her performance in drawing the tree and printing the alphabet a few minutes later after she was neutralized.

Since Dr. Lee shared his discovery of the neutralizing symptom-relieving technique with us, hundreds of thousands of neutralizing doses of extracts and/or solutions prepared from foods, chemicals, tobacco smoke, house dust, pollens, molds, etc., have been given to thousands of patients in the throes of allergic reactions, and in many instances almost miraculously their symptoms of headache, nausea, fatigue, depression, arthritis, asthma, etc. have disappeared.

A Nonpsychiatric Approach to Psychosomatic Disorders and Mental Problems

Dr. Theron G. Randolph of Chicago and Zion, Illinois, is my highly respected friend, colleague, and mentor. His work has permanently affected the primary direction of modern medicine. I hardly know where to start a list of his accomplishments, for he is one of the outstanding investigators in clinical ecology and it was his work that led me to the concept of bio-ecologic diseases. His term "ecologic mental illness" will someday be familiar to everyone; he coined this designation to describe the numerous types of mental illness he has shown to be the result of malfunctions in the brain due to food, beverage, dust, dander, pollen, and chemical allergies.

Dr. Randolph is the premier investigator of a nonpsychiatric approach to mental illness, irritability, and behavior problems in children, allergic headache, depression from home exposures to gas and combustion products of gas and oil, addictive eating as a cause of obesity, food addiction leading to alcoholism, allergic fatigue, acute episodes of psychotic behavior due to allergy (with motion picture film documentation), allergic disorders of the intestinal tract, house dust allergy, etc. The list is long and revelatory, his published papers numbering well over one hundred. The contents of many of Dr. Randolph's papers will be discussed throughout this book.

Internal Allergies Caused by Dust, Molds, and Pollens

I have included my work here with that of my colleagues because I have been able to treat many problem cases successfully as a direct result of my research into the area of internal sensitivities to dust, molds, pollens, and animal danders. I have found that any of the common species of mold present in the home or outdoors is capable of producing many different kinds of internal symptoms not previously recognized as being due to allergy. Traditional, conventionally trained allergists still employ less reliable skin tests to diagnose allergy to molds, as well as dust, animal danders, pollens, and foods. In testing for mold allergy, they are searching for the causes of symptoms that affect the membrane surfaces of the eyes, nose, throat, sinuses, and bronchial tubes. If the patient does not react to the skin tests for mold allergy, he or she is usually considered to be unaffected by these very potent environmental substances. If, on the other hand, the conventional allergist notes the appearance of positive skin tests, he will then usually treat the patient for the molds that caused reactions on the patient's skin.

Dr. Harris Hosen of Port Arthur, Texas, who introduced me to the technique of nasal inhalation testing—"sniff" tests—has performed thousands of such tests on his patients and found that sniff tests are far more accurate than the old-fashioned intradermal scratch tests. About fifteen years ago, I repeated Dr. Hosen's work and was able to confirm and extend his observations. An outstanding example of the inaccuracy of skin testing along traditional lines is exemplified by one of my asthmatic patients. I obtained twelve positive skin tests in this patient when I tested her with extracts prepared from twelve different molds. I also obtained a series of negative skin tests with other mold extracts. When I gave her small amounts of powdered molds to inhale from the end of a toothpick, her reaction to these direct bronchial challenges were a revelation to me because only *one* of the twelve skin-test positive molds, a mold called *alternaria,* caused her to have an attack of asthma. The second important surprise was my discovery that stemphyllium, a mold that had been largely ignored in allergy at that time, was negative on skin testing and yet a sniff test for it gave her a more severe attack of asthma than the sniff test with alternaria had. She also had an asthmatic attack when given the sniff test with house dust.*

As I thought about this aspect of allergy, I was able to make another contribution to bio-ecologic medicine: I realized that if any inhaled allergens, such as dust, molds, pollens, insect particles, etc., became trapped in the mucus secretions that cover the surfaces of the nose and throat, these inhaled substances would then be swallowed with the mucus and treated by the stomach and intestine as any type of food or beverage that was digested and then absorbed into the bloodstream. A substance entering the bloodstream would be circulated throughout the body reaching all tissues, including the brain. In addition, some small particles that enter the lungs might be acted upon by the normal secretions in the bronchial tubes and be absorbed into the lung circulation in lesser quantities. Thus in two fashions nasal inhalants can expose the entire body to a whole spectrum of allergic symptoms far beyond simple hives, runny noses, and difficult breathing.

*As I continued testing patients with dusts, molds, pollens and animal danders by inhalation testing, I was able to induce headaches, depression, itching of the skin, abdominal pain, weakness, and mental confusion. These experiences with nasal inhalation testing gave me conclusive evidence of the inaccuracy of skin tests. And treatment can only be effective when the diagnosis is correct!

3
Physical and Mental Allergies in Adults

Are Physical Ailments Allergic Symptoms?

Countless times in the millions of tests my colleagues and I have performed, patients' chronic physical miseries have been shown to have their origins in allergic responses. My first experience with physical symptoms as a direct reaction to an allergy took place about fifteen years ago. I remember it well because it completely changed the direction and scope of my practice, and nearly frightened me to death at the same time:

CASE STUDY: COLITIS/HOARSENESS

The patient, Martha D., was a very pleasant lady who particularly liked to sing in her church choir, but something was affecting her voice so that she wasn't always able to sing to the best of her ability. At this stage in my medical career, I had just become familiar with the work of physicians like Drs. Theron Randolph, Herbert Rinkel, and Carleton Lee, and I thought I should investigate food allergy as a possible cause of her problems with her vocal cords and nasal passages. Her initial course of treatments with weekly injections of dust, mold, and pollen extracts combined with a respiratory bacterial vaccine had helped her considerably, but there was room for improvement. We sought the extra clearing of symptoms that would, hopefully, restore her voice to its normal tonal quality and keep it there.

Knowing that it is often a patient's favorite food to which the patient is allergic, I tested her first for milk allergy because she had told me that she loved milk and drank it "constantly." Within minutes after testing her for possible respiratory tract allergy to milk, her nose began to drip and then became totally blocked, giving her voice a deep nasal quality.

We were both very excited about this discovery. She was happy that we obviously had found an important factor that had a major effect on her voice; and I was elated because with my very first provocative test to determine the presence of allergic sensitivity to foods, I had found one, and I had been been able to select the offending food so easily and accurately by reviewing her dietary habits. I told Mrs. D. that I wanted to watch her reaction run its course and that I would return to the testing room in a few minutes to follow her milk reaction.

I was in another part of the office with another patient when I heard Mrs. D. cry out, "Doctor! Please come quickly—something terrible is happening!"

At that moment, with her frightened voice resounding down the corridors of my clinic, and fully aware of the fact that I probably was the only physician east of the Mississippi River doing this kind of controversial food testing, my heart sank to meet my stomach and my knees became a little weak. Mustering as much combined haste and restraint as possible to keep from mowing down patients and nurses alike in the hall, and to maintain what I then conceived to be a doctorlike decorum, I walked rapidly down the hall and into her test cubicle.

She was definitely in a very upset condition, breathing rapidly, her eyes big, and she was obviously very frightened. I had, to put it mildly, a concern that I might have done something harmful to this person who trusted me and had come to me to be helped. Then, all of my previous training paid off and the doctor in me came to the fore. I looked at her with clinical objectivity. Even though she was breathing rapidly, her color was good, she was able to stand up, and she could talk; she was alert, well oriented, and her eyes were bright. Her major body functions were normal when I examined her chest, pulse, and blood pressure. Her heart and lungs were working a little harder than usual but her pulse was strong, her blood pressure was normal, and she was in excellent contact with her surroundings. So I knew, with a feeling of great relief, that I had not precipitated the allergists' worst fear, anaphylactic shock—a life-threatening, acute reaction brought on by administration of treatment material. She obviously was having what is generally described as an anxiety attack. Once I was completely satisfied that she was not in any danger at all I instructed my nurses to make sure that she was all right and to look in on her in the testing room every few minutes. I told Mrs. D. that I would be back to check on her condition every five minutes or so. On my third or fourth visit, when I asked how she felt, she complained of severe right abdominal pains, but her feelings of anxiety had disappeared completely.

I took her to an examining room to check her abdomen and detected a spasm of her right ascending colon. I asked her if she had ever had this kind of pain in this area before. She stated that for many years she had had recurring episodes of abdominal pain that would go on for three or four weeks and then culminate in an attack of bloody diarrhea. She would be all right for four to six weeks and then the pain-diarrhea cycle would be repeated again. She had consulted a gastroenterologist on the faculty at Yale Medical School. After his examination, including X-rays, he somehow concluded that she had spastic colitis due to emotional problems. She told me she had been placed on a series of unsuccessful diets to control her condition; her current diet was a bland one with a great deal of milk and dairy products in it.

By means of retesting and elimination, I was able to demonstrate that with the best of intentions her physician had prescribed a milk-rich diet, which was exactly what was causing her problems! He was totally unaware of the important role of food allergy (beyond the "if it bothers you, don't eat it anymore" stage). I asked her why she hadn't mentioned her gastrointestinal troubles, the pain and bloody diarrhea, that had been going on for years. Her answer was, "But you are my *allergist!*" She had given me the information that she believed an allergist should have as she perceived the specialty of allergy.

About one-third of the allergies for which I tested her did cause difficulties. I was so excited by my experience with this patient and the gamut of reactions induced by testing that I contacted a psychiatrist friend of mine, Dr. Gilbert Rose, of the Yale University Medical School Department of Psychiatry, and asked him to join me in performing a "double blind" allergy study with this patient in my office. I wanted an opportunity to demonstrate the effects of food allergy and, in Dr. Rose, I would have a devil's advocate in the form of a psychiatrist as a participant in the study.

It was important that the design of the study be completely objective: I took various extracts and grouped them on the desk for Dr. Rose. The "control" was sterile salt water (saline); in another group I had the extracts of foods to which Mrs. D. had not reacted; in a third group were the foods to which she had reacted. Dr. Rose's and my plan was that while I was out of the room, he would place a food extract known only to him in a syringe, record the identity of the test material, and hand the syringe to me when I entered the room. Mrs. D. and I would have no knowledge of what was in the syringe. (The appearance of the test solutions varied from clear to light, yellow to light brown, and there was no possible way to identify the contents of the syringe.) I would give her an injection of an unknown test substance (unknown to me and the patient) and leave the room. Dr. Rose would set a timer to ring in twenty minutes and remain in the testing room with Mrs. D. She was to describe in detail any subjective symptoms she might experience, and he would make objective observations of any reactions that occurred: changes in her voice, mental state (affect), behavior, facial expressions; whether she was pale or flushed, whether she seemed tired, her eyes bright or glazed; the position of her body —whether she was slumped, sitting up, or leaning on the examining table or against the wall.

At the end of the afternoon, Dr. Rose and I reviewed the results of our investigation. He told me that the salt water (the control test solution) produced no symptoms, but that milk and yeast caused many of her commonly experienced physical and mental symptoms. Dr. Rose and I were intrigued by our findings and wanted to share this newfound information with our colleagues because we realized that we had made some very important observations. We wrote a paper we called "Emotional Reactions Precipitated by Allergens" and were much disappointed that no psychiatry or psychology journals would accept it. So we changed the title of our paper in order to make it more acceptable: "May Emotional Reactions Be Precipitated by Allergens?" The new title would not raise the hackles of the doctors steeped in established medical concepts, and we would indicate that there might be some question regarding our observations and conclusions—even though there was no question in our minds, since we had proved them by established and acceptable medical test standards. The editor of the *Connecticut State Medical Journal* accepted our paper for publication; it was the first article of its kind in medical literature.

Very excited by my experience with food-related respiratory allergy in this patient, I performed food and chemical tests on subsequent patients who came to me with classical allergies in order to determine what roles foods and chemicals might play in asthma, hay fever, sinus conditions, hives, etc. I conducted tests in most of those cases, and in many I found symptoms present in other parts of their bodies which, upon questioning, I was told were problems from which they had always suffered and for which they had never been able to find a cause.

One lady with asthma was tested for cereal grain sensitivities, and when she was exposed to corn extract she developed pain in her left ankle. When I asked her if she had ever experienced pain of this type before, she replied (a little indignantly), "Of course, that's my arthritis." I asked her if she had it any place else. She said, "No, just in my ankle." I practically jumped from behind my desk with excitement. I asked, "Do you realize what we have just done? We have reproduced your chronic arthritis pain with a test for allergy to corn, and corn is present in your daily diet in many forms: in the corn flakes cereal you are eating each morning, in the corn oil you use to cook, in the cornstarch that thickens gravy, in the corn sweeter (dextrose or glucose) that is in canned fruit." After she removed corn in all forms from her diet, her "arthritis" disappeared.

CASE STUDY: MULTIPLE SCLEROSIS/MIGRAINE HEADACHES/
FATIGUE

Mrs. Sally Storm (her real name is given here with her permission) is a middle-aged woman who lives in Weston, Connecticut. She came to my office in November 1976 for headaches that had been present for more than twenty years.

The headaches were of several types: one would start at the back of her neck and shoot upward and forward. The other was a migraine, which began in the right temple and was sharply localized as if daggers were stabbing her. Many times she would have nausea and vomiting along with a pinching sensation in the upper border of her right ear; her right eye would turn quite red and tear, and her nose would become stuffy. Her third type of headache occurred in the forehead and was related to her hormone balance; it would appear a few days before her menstrual period or sometimes in the middle of her cycle. This kind of headache would disappear with aspirin.

Mrs. Storm also had a limp. Her condition was diagnosed as multiple sclerosis (MS) by the Department of Neurology at Yale Medical School. This is how Mrs. Storm described her limp to me during our first consultation: "My limping often varies in severity. On some days it is very bad, on other days it is greatly reduced and is much better." In other words, her MS symptoms had a very special characteristic in that the intensity of her limp changed greatly and rapidly during the course of a single day. Her doctors at Yale told her that the MS would "just have to run its course." The daily variations in her MS symptomatology were not recognized as having any real clinical importance.

The evening before she came to the office for her first visit, she had been "terribly weak" and walked with considerable difficulty. However, by morning she was feeling much stronger and she could walk much better. My immediate conclusion was that she could not yet possibly have very much permanent neurologic damage in the sense that she had "sclerosed" areas of her spinal cord. Sclerosis in MS means that some nerve tissue has been permanently damaged and scarred; an area of sclerosis would be an area of scar tissue. So if she had multiple sclerotic areas, they were not going to disappear and she should not be better some days and worse on others. And she certainly should not be getting better and worse during the course of a few hours on the same day—permanently damaged areas in the spinal cord just don't function that way.

Her case fascinated me. One of my key signs that an allergy or allergylike condition due to external factors may be present is the *reversibility* of symptoms. If Mrs. Storm was limping one day and better the next, it seemed to me that her MS symptoms could possibly be responses to some thing(s) she was eating, drinking, or with which she was coming into contact. After all, if a person has a rather severe nasal allergy to cat dander and gets a heavy exposure to a cat, the person's nose will probably itch or sneeze considerably, and then may develop a profuse discharge and/or become "all clogged up." When either the person or the cat goes away, the aforementioned symptoms will begin to clear up. Certainly something was happening in Mrs. Storm's nervous system that was very uncharacteristic of the permanent form of spinal cord scarring that is present in the advanced states of MS where there are no longer any remissions.

Mrs. Storm told me that her illness began at about the same time she moved into her present home in 1963. Because the house was not a new building, I suspected that there might be something about the house itself that was directly involved in the causation of her MS. Perhaps it had been chemically treated in some manner: Maybe it had been treated for termites with creosote, or contaminated with very long acting insect- or pest-exterminating chemicals; or it was possible that there was a high concentration of nerve-damaging molds from a dampness problem or an abundance of potted plants;* or perhaps the house-

---

*My investigations of major forms of reversible injury due to common environmental factors responsible for serious physical and mental disorders have shown that molds, house dust, animal danders, and pollen can be to blame. (Molds are especially potent incitants of nervous system disorders in my experience). All physicians know that various antibiotics derived from different kinds of streptomyces molds can cause permanent deafness due to permanent injury to the nerve that goes from the brain to the ears—the eighth cranial nerve. If the mold-derived drug is stopped in time, the early phase of deafness may not become permanent. Chest physicians are well acquainted with the fact that

hold air was polluted with gas fumes from the heating system. Mrs. Storm also gave me a history of chronic eczema from early childhood which eventually cleared in her teens, and she indicated that thyroid treatment was believed to have eventually cured the eczema. Of course, eczema is a term that is very widely used to describe a variety of chronic skin conditions, but her condition could well have been the allergic eczema of childhood, and it gave just one more possible clue that she might be an allergic person.

About one-half of the tests that my technicians performed on Mrs. Storm caused no reactions whatsoever. This large group of negative tests served as a series of controls, which are an important aspect of many kinds of testing.

The following information is taken from my technicians' notes describing the patient's responses to tests:

Egg: The middle of her back and the back of her neck felt a little sensitive. She described this as being as if the circulation had improved in those areas.

Coffee: She became slightly nervous and moderately tense, with difficulty in concentrating. Then she felt "spaced out." When most patients use this expression it means that things appear to be unreal. It was an effort for her to maintain contact with her surroundings. Next, she had some mild tingling within her lower extremity, which was a familiar symptom to her; it seemed to me that this might be important because it was the leg that she limped with. This coffee test suggested the possibility that some aspect of her MS and limp could be related to the ingestion of coffee.

Milk: Her right ear began to hurt, and she developed a mild headache. (These were familiar symptoms.)

Wheat: She had a slight feeling of tension in the right side of her head.

Baker's yeast: She felt frightened, and her heart rate increased slightly.

Orange: She felt moderately stimulated and then became very restless. She was very much aware of what she referred to as her circulation, but she could not describe her response as being any-

---

Seromycin can cause psychotic behavior and convulsions when this antibiotic is employed in tuberculosis treatment. Chloromycetin has an effect on brain tissue that can cause a period of mental depression. Molds produce potent by-products.

thing more than that. I told her to eliminate orange from her diet for a few months and then eat an orange to see if she could tolerate it.

Honey: She became moderately tired with honey, which she used frequently as a sweetener.

Oats: She had weakness in her legs and tenderness at the base of her spine. And this also was a familiar feeling. This test was done because her diet included this cereal grain, a member of the grass family. It is present in oatmeal, oatmeal cookies, and granola.

Cane sugar: She became extremely restless, very uneasy, and said, "This is my worst reaction so far."

Lettuce: She developed stuffiness in her left nostril, and her left leg became very tingly. (Coffee caused mild tingling.)

Regular house dust: She had uneasiness in both legs, tightness in the back of her neck, and a generalized feeling of uneasiness.

Mixed grass pollens: A prickly sensation developed in the top of her head, her legs felt wiggly and restless.

Chlorine: She became slightly sleepy at first, with tenderness in her upper spine. Her head felt heavy. Next, she felt as though she were quite "high," as if she were drunk.

House dust from Endo Laboratory: Tightness developed in the back of her neck, and she became a little sleepy.

Ethanol: She became a little sleepy. (This is Dr. Randolph's petroleum alcohol chemical test.)

Weed pollens: Her typical respiratory and cerebral symptoms were brought on. She sneezed twice, developed a runny nose, and became sleepy.

Rice: This made her moderately sleepy with a tightness in the back of her neck

Onions: She became sleepy with one dose and then became restless with another. (We usually give test materials in three, four, or more different doses.)

Food preservative mixture: Tenderness appeared down her spine, her head felt a bit stuffy, and she could not think very clearly.

Auto exhaust: She felt tingling in the left leg—the site of her MS.

Lysol: She became sleepy. (For my final testing dose, the greatest strength of Lysol that I used was a solution the manufacturer said was safe to employ in washing a baby's crib. It was my conclusion that a solution that was shown to be safe for a baby's crib, and we all know that babies lick their cribs, certainly would have to be considered safe. A rather similar line of reasoning is followed in the preparation and use of various types of fruit and vegetable insecticide spray materials.)

Mushrooms (which are related to molds): She became slightly sleepy.

Yellow food coloring: No reaction.

Fruit tree spray: A slight tension occurred in the back of her neck and she became sleepy. Here again we have a familiar pattern of symptoms.

Spinach: No reaction.

Peanuts: She felt spaced out and mentally sluggish.

Tuna fish: She became a little sleepy.

Mixed vegetable gums (used in candy making): She was a little sleepy and had mild palpitations.

Potatoes: Negative.

Corn: Negative.

Celery: Negative.

Pecan: She became sleepy.

Estrogen: This gave her a moderate, dull headache in the right side of her head, extending into her ear.

Apricot: Her eyelids felt a little heavy, and she became a little sleepy.

Rye: Negative.

Garlic: Negative.

Sole: Negative.

Influenza (flu) vaccine: This gave her a mild headache in the right frontal area. (Flu virus is toxic to the nervous system.)

Vegetable garden spray: Tightness developed in the upper chest, and she fell asleep. When she awoke she asked us not to give her the other dose.

Penicillium (mold): Her eyelids became very heavy and very itchy, and she became very sleepy.

Monilia (mold): She was very sleepy, dopy, not alert. Monilia lives on the skin and in the bowels. It often causes a very uncomfortable form of vaginal inflammation and infection.

Aspergillis (mold): Her right upper leg felt stimulated and "sensitive," and she had a need to wiggle it all the time. Then the right foot became numb. Even though the MS limp was localized only in the left leg, something important seemed to be taking place in the yet uninvolved right lower extremity.

Alternaria (mold): She became moderately restless. (This is a very common mold.)

Hormodendrum (mold): This made her sleepy, then quite restless.

Phoma (mold): Her right foot became numb. She described it as being "asleep."

Pullularia (mold): She felt a little spaced out, very sleepy, flushed, warm. Her eyelids felt very heavy, indicating that there were test-related changes in the circulation of her head, because we changed the color of her face by affecting its blood supply. As the facial blood supply was increased because of dilated (relaxed) blood vessels, some of the blood vessels supplying her brain may have constricted, reducing the oxygen and blood sugar levels to the brain.

Stemphyllium (mold): She became very sleepy, her right leg became numb, and there was a dull ache in the back of her head.

Trichophyton (mold): No reaction.

Fusarium (mold): This gave her a headache, then she became slightly sleepy. She sneezed once and developed a runny nose.

Helminthosporium (mold): The back of her neck became a bit stiff, and she got a little sleepy.

Mrs. Storm is on Dr. Herbert Rinkel's Rotary Diversified Diet, and I am also giving her injection treatments of food extracts for food allergy. She has a newfound feeling of well-being and her entire outlook on life has improved. On July 9, 1977, with a great sense of personal satisfaction, I recorded on Mrs. Storm's chart that she told me, "I am very excited. My children say I am walking better than they have seen me walk in years!"

The simple but generally overlooked fact that her MS symptoms came and went had a great impact on me. This I believed was a major clue that a form of allergy might be, at least, a contributing factor at the root of some of her problems. Happily, this time I was right. She did not have to "let the disease of MS run its course," as advised by her consulting neurologist. We could do something in this case, and we did.

CASE STUDY: MIGRAINE/FATIGUE/DIARRHEA

"I have very little faith in doctors" was one of the first statements a new patient, Celeste R., made to me. I was not offended or shocked. I have heard these unhappy words many times from other patients during their first consultation with me.

Celeste's major complaints at age forty-seven were migraine headaches, chronic fatigue, and diarrhea. Headaches and diarrhea started at age thirty-five, fatigue had been present about two years, and for the past year and a half the diarrhea had been getting worse. When she came to me she was under psychiatric care. Her psychiatrist stated that these symptoms were due to emotional causes which he believed he had been able to trace back to her childhood. As a young girl she had been bedridden for seven years.

Her previous doctors had overlooked a very important characteristic time-and-symptom pattern in this case, and they also ignored her numerous observations concerning the effects of foods and alcohol on her health. Her migraine headaches (always in the left side of her head, and associated with nausea and vomiting) would regularly appear at 6:00 PM with a severe pain in her left eye "like a knife sticking in." This was the pattern for eleven years.

In addition to that pattern, she also knew if she took one drink of rye whisky, the next day—"almost like clockwork"—she would get a severe headache, but not her typical migraine.

Her abnormal bowel movements also followed a definite time pattern: Every night between 8:00 and 9:00 PM she would have an episode of diarrhea related to her evening meal. She knew that many foods caused her to become nauseated. Milk made her nauseous, and she often had to go to bed to rest because the nausea was so severe that it was impossible for her to function. When she drank as little as one ounce of tea, she became nauseous. Lettuce produced nausea, and she would experience a repeating of the taste of lettuce in her mouth for several hours. Tomato, cheese, mayonnaise, vinegar, and orange juice also made her nauseous.

One hard-boiled egg was tolerated, but two eggs produced nausea. Wheat flour in a meat juice to thicken gravy also made her nauseous.

Although she had been avoiding most of the foods that she knew made her ill, it was clear there were other foods she was eating that also caused her trouble; she had moderately severe upper abdominal cramping and would feel "very full" after each meal.

She had made a series of important observations that indicated she also was addicted to some food or foods. If she did not eat on schedule—if she was only fifteen minutes late for a meal— she would become mentally confused, unable to concentrate, and would develop a tremor of her hands that caused her to drop things at home and in the office. "If I eat a sandwich, I feel better." But the sandwich always was made with rye bread and lettuce, and it would contain either beef or pork or chicken.

She also knew she had some chemical sensitivities. She noted when she was exposed to tobacco smoke, varnish, shellac, or the fumes of paint, she would get a severe nonmigraine headache. Scented deodorants, air freshener, hair and scented sprays would also produce a headache. Gasoline would give pains in the lower forehead in the region of her frontal sinuses. If she was exposed to truck or bus exhaust fumes, she got "uncomfortable and quite dizzy." Detergents would give her a brief episode of shortness of breath and sneezing.

After taking a comprehensive chronologic bio-ecologically oriented history of her condition, I transferred her to the technicians in the testing section of the center. The following are some selected examples of the kinds of reactions she had to tests with drops of food extracts, dust, mold and pollen extracts, and chemical solutions placed under her tongue for rapid absorption into her system.

Automobile exhaust: She had generalized itching, severe stomach cramps, and extreme nausea.

Natural gas: (She had a gas stove in her apartment.) When testing with this material we usually use a series of four progressively increasing doses of the natural gas solutions. After the second dose, she developed a moderately severe headache, saying, "This is the beginning of a migraine." We did not wish to make her more uncomfortable than necessary to establish a diagnosis and we discontinued the test at this time.

Mixture of food preservatives: She developed severe nausea, irritability, and fatigue. She had moderate shortness of breath and felt extremely hot.

All-purpose plant, flower, vegetable, and tree spray: She had severe chest pain, nausea, and a moderate headache around her left eye and the top of her head that changed to her typical migraine. We stopped the test.

Sole: There was pain in her left eye.

Black pepper: She had head pain, nausea, and the familiar sensation of fullness in her abdomen.

Peaches: (She loved them and always had a supply of them). She had mild heart palpitations and severe generalized itching.

Baker's yeast: She had difficulty breathing, with a sensation that she couldn't breathe well and not enough air was getting into her chest. She developed pain in her left thigh and moderate pain in the left side of her head. She asked that we stop the test because she felt she was going to have a migraine.

This reaction was caused by the first dose of baker's yeast, and she was observed carefully to see if the test-provoked symptoms were going to clear or persist. (Of course, if the symptoms from any test are severe, we neutralize the reaction with the technique explained on page 36, and I make a judgment as to whether or not the symptoms a patient is experiencing are of sufficient interest to be filmed or taped for future reference.) Ten minutes after her reaction developed (we hadn't neutralized her symptoms) she said that she felt "strange." Suddenly, the cup she was holding fell to the floor; she had completely forgotten, or was unaware, that she had a cup in her hand.

Rye: (Remember, she always had rye-bread sandwiches): She sneezed and felt some pressure in her chest.

Milk: She developed nausea and a mild migraine in the left side of her head.

Lettuce (Remember, she was also eating lettuce every day in her sandwiches): She got a sharp pain above her left eye and felt a need to have more air get into her chest. She became aware of her heart beating, and when we examined her, the pulse rate had increased six beats per minute.

Beef (She recalled doctors had wanted her to "build herself up" during childhood, and she was fed a great deal of beef. The habit of eating beef frequently continued throughout her life): The beef caused pains in her forehead and numbness in her left arm and left leg. She had some difficulty breathing, accompanied by a sensation of heaviness in her chest.

Dust mites (particles of a microscopic insect that are one of the major components of house dust): She developed severe nausea with the first dose and requested we discontinue the test.

Alternaria (mold): She had nausea, moderate pain in the left side of her chest and arm, and moderate difficulty in breathing.

Stemphyllium (mold): She had a severe headache for thirty seconds, which then decreased in intensity to one of moderate severity.

Hormodendrum (mold): She experienced a slight difficulty in breathing and felt as if her head would "float away." Very dark circles (allergic "shiners") appeared under her eyes, and this area also became very puffy. (It is not unusual for my technicians and me to observe areas of puffiness and changes—darkening or fading—in allergic "shiners" as seen in this patient. I have seen the joints of arthritic patients swell up, become red and painful during the course of a test. We have had a number of severe, almost instant episodes of abdominal bloating with visible distention. The stomach of one man who was tested with potato extract became so distended within a few minutes that he actually looked about seven months' pregnant. During testing some people have complained that their clothing is too tight; they have had to open their belts and adjust their skirts. Several of my female patients have at least two sizes of clothing in their wardrobes for this reason. During some tests rings and shoes become tight.)

Mucor (mold): She had moderate pains in her left arm and left wrist and a heavy sensation in her chest. (A reaction of this type could easily be misinterpreted as a possible heart attack. There are unrecognized allergic people who have been frightened that they are having a heart attack because of allergic chest, neck, jaw, shoulder, arm, and waist pain. It isn't a heart attack—the chest examination is negative and nothing shows up on the chest X-rays and cardiogram.

Phoma (mold): She developed slight nausea, itching of the eyes, pain in her left arm, and her face became flushed. (The subject of facial flushing is of interest to me because it is a form of objective evidence, which in most instances is accompanied by nonobjective symptoms. Not only do we have subjective evidence in that the patient tells us how she feels during the course of a reaction to a test, but it is apparent to all observers that the patient has become flushed. Flushing and pallor are often caused by allergy, and flushing during testing is a clear indication that a state of allergic sensitivity is responsible for an increase in the flow of blood to the face. An allergic reaction can increase or decrease the flow of blood to the face through its effects on any of the blood vessels that carry oxygen and other essential substances. Allergy can, and certainly does, also have the capacity to affect the blood vessels supplying the inner portion of the head, and this includes that all-important and highly complicated living computer with a fantastic memory bank, the human brain.

(Allergic spasm or dilation of important arteries in the head that supply the brain can have major effects on all of the functions of the brain. In addition to allergic influence on the blood supply to the brain, there are many environmental substances that may have direct effect on various groups of brain cells after they enter the body by ingestion or respiration. Very often it is subjective complaints and reversible physical disorders that bring patients to their doctors. That's why I want to emphasize again that the patient, his spouse or parents are our best sources of information. We believe our patients; they have all the facts and want to help and be helped.)

After Celeste had completed testing based on her history and probable exposures, it was easy for me to understand many of her symptoms. Although she was on a very limited diet, she continued to have some symptoms after every meal. How could anyone be well with all her allergies? Almost all of the foods she was eating bothered her to some extent; she was the type of patient whom Dr. Randolph has identified as being a "universal food reactor." She would have been in serious difficulty for the rest of her life, and it is probable that she would have become progressively worse with the passage of time, if no one had ever investigated her for bodywide allergies to foods and inhalants and chemical sensitivities.

Also, because she reacted to many of the environmental substances for which we tested her, I began to suspect that those seven years she was bedridden could have been allergy-related to some degree. Remember, she was on a program of bed rest and she was highly allergic. Could there possibly have been a tragic misdiagnosis of TB, or could she have had an illness that was made worse because of a serious underlying allergic disorder that was present at the same time?

This was not a hopeless case by any means. Once I determined the particular spectrum of offending foods, beverages, airborne particles, and environmental chemicals to which she was sensitive and reacting, it was possible for us to help her. We began by using Dr. Herbert Rinkel's Rotary Diversified Diet principle and selected a diet for her in which she ate the foods to which she was only mildly allergic on a five-day rotation, with three different foods each day. (Just following a rotary diet alone will often be enough to give considerable relief to many allergic individuals.) We supervised her environmental clean-up program to get rid of the airborne particles and household chemical agents that had been affecting her health for years. She also began a series of allergic desensitization treatments for unavoidable airborne allergens.

In her follow-up consultation several months after treatment had been started, she stated that she definitely felt much better. The diarrhea was now reduced in severity and frequency; it occurred only every seven to ten days. Her migraine headaches (so bad she had said that she "would lie in bed hoping she would die because of the pain") were much less frequent and these were not of as long duration as before. They lasted only one or two hours, usually one. The former prolonged bouts of severe and incapacitating nausea were reduced in intensity and duration. When I last spoke to her she said, "Doctor, this is the first time in my illness that I have made any progress whatsoever."

CASE STUDY: EPILEPSY

A sixteen-year-old girl who had been having epileptic seizures for several months was seen by my fellow ecologist Lawrence D. Dickey, MD, a past president of the Society for Clinical Ecology. During the course of his consultation with her, he asked which food she would miss most if it was eliminated from her diet. "Iced tea" was her immediate reply.

For a year she had been drinking iced tea every day, taking this beverage from two to four times per day. Tea was eliminated from her diet for a period of four days, and she participated in a deliberate ingestion test for possible sensitivity to tea on the fifth day. She had a seizure in twenty minutes. Her heightened reaction to tea after abstaining from this nonnutritive beverage for four days is an excellent demonstration of Dr. Herbert Rinkel's original observations with which he formulated the deliberate feeding test which is an important diagnostic aspect of his Rotary Diversified Diet.

Dr. Theron G. Randolph has emphasized the fact that while there are difficulties, sometimes quite serious, in making a specific diagnosis in cases of epilepsy, a major effort should be made for each person who is so afflicted. He further believes that the neurologist has an ethical responsibility to diagnose, if possible, the underlying *causes* of his epileptic patients' seizures: He should not limit his diagnostic efforts to the currently employed methods of investigating and medicating cases of convulsive disorders. A homebound epileptic with a severe form of this illness is probably receiving high doses of anticonvulsant drugs, which may keep him quite drowsy and unable to participate in either social, pleasurable, or productive activities. Furthermore, such an individual probably requires a great deal of supervision, and this places an additional burden on the family since someone—a relative or a hired employee—must always be available. A carefully supervised diagnostic evaluation in an in-hospital ecologic unit is the right of every human being whose epileptic condition could possibly be better controlled with less or *no* mind-clouding medications. A comprehensive bio-ecologically oriented program of physiologically sound measures to control the identifiable causes of each case of epilepsy should be available to every individual who can benefit from such care. *Skilled prescribing of potent drugs is not enough!*

CASE STUDY: HEART DISEASE

Dr. Joseph Harkavy, former chief of the Allergy Clinic at Mount Sinai Hospital in New York, former president of the New York Allergy Society, and vice-president of the American Academy of Allergy, has published remarkable electrocardiograms of a young man which were taken while he was having an allergic reaction to coffee. His EKG tracing had changes in it that were indistinguishable from those associated with coronary occlusion. (This type of heart attack is due to an obstructed coronary artery which supplies oxygen and nourishment to the heart muscle itself.) When this patient was given an antihistamine or an injection of adrenalin, his electrocardiogram returned to normal. What most probably had occurred was that there had been a constricting allergic spasm of the ring of muscles in the wall of the coronary vessel. This caused a decreased flow of blood, which led to decreased oxygen and nutrition to the tissues in a particular region of his heart, which resulted in the EKG changes characteristic of coronary occlusion.

I believe that some people have heart attacks that are caused by food and chemical allergy. Allergists know that when many reversible allergic reactions occur repeatedly in the same patient, there may be some permanent damage or weakening of the particular organ or system involved. Eventually there may be some serious kind of breakdown following these allergic attacks. For example, in some cases of long-standing bronchial asthma, the walls of the bronchial tubes become thickened, causing some degree of permanent lung obstruction. With respect to food allergy as a factor in some type of heart attacks, it seems important to note that some people have suffered from "acute indigestion" before and/or along with their heart attacks. A heart attack may be associated with typical food allergy symptoms such as nausea, vomiting, or other gastrointestinal disturbances.

What if some of these people had acute allergic muscle-con-stricting spasms of the muscles in the walls of their main coro-nary artery? This artery is the lifeline that sustains the muscular walls of the heart, which is really a form of muscular blood pump. An allergic coronary spasm can greatly reduce the flow of blood in this indispensable blood vessel. Suppose the allergy-caused spasm wasn't relieved and this allowed a blood clot to form in the now more slowly moving blood of an already diseased coronary artery behind this area of spasm. Suddenly, in the midst of a prolonged allergic reaction, an obstructing, heart-damaging, and life-threatening blood clot might form and —disaster!

I have induced numerous episodes of chest pains during the course of testing patients who had been carefully examined by specialists and pronounced to be free of heart disease. My col-leagues and I have also caused chest pain in some patients who were diagnosed as having heart disease, some of whom had been having frequent chest pains over a long period of time.

About four years ago a man brought his wife to the office for me to investigate her long-standing complaints of headache, fatigue, depression, and "upset stomach." When the husband saw how I was able to reproduce and identify the cause of his wife's symptoms, he asked if I would perform some tests on him.

When we tested him for possible allergy to a number of foods, including his favorite, milk, we reproduced his typical chest ("heart") pains with milk extract. I advised him to eliminate milk immediately in all forms, including milk products like butter, cheese, ice cream, etc., for at least three weeks. He followed my instructions, and he was completely free of the frightening chest pains that his internist could not diagnose. I told my patient that he could obtain additional proof that milk allergy had been causing the chest pain by taking a deliberate milk-feeding test, which consisted of drinking a few tall glasses of milk and eating some cottage cheese and some ice cream. And he was to then wait to see what might happen. Within minutes after he took this dietary challenge, he had his usual "heart" pains back again. A diagnostic flareup was produced due to a state of heightened sensitivity to milk after a period of milk avoidance.

This man did not have the usual kind of heart disease. But he lived in constant fear that a serious heart attack was just a matter of time. All he had to do for the present was eliminate milk and milk products, and he probably would be fine. If he were to go on a rotary diet, he could perhaps learn how much better he might be able to feel and which additional foods, if any, affected his health in other ways. Dr. Harkavy, author of *Vascular Allergy and Its Systemic Manifestations,* pointed out, "With increasing knowledge of hypersensitivity it becomes apparent that certain specific tissues may become involved in the allergic response, in conjunction with or to the exclusion of those of the respiratory tract. Information already available has indicated that sensitization to exogenous (external, environmental) factors, such as tobacco, foods, drugs, antibiotics and infection may account not only for reversible, but also for irreversible reactions in the heart and blood vessels."

CASE STUDY: CARDIAC NEUROSIS

Patty J., a woman in her thirties whom I saw early in my development as a bio-ecologist, was referred to me by her internist for evaluation of a chronic sinus condition. It turned out that the sinus problem was the least important of the disorders that I was able to solve for her. Without any awareness of her many other physical and "emotional" disorders, I proceeded to duplicate an amazing assortment of physical and mental symptoms that were very familiar to her and totally unanticipated by me.

Her personal physician was an internist with a special interest in cardiology, and after a thorough study, he had come to the conclusion that her frequent episodes of tachycardia (rapid heart rate) associated with mental depression were manifestations of a "cardiac neurosis" and referred her to a psychiatrist. From the bio-ecologically oriented history that I belatedly obtained, I was able to prove that her tachycardia was not a "cardiac neurosis," it was a manifestation of cardiac susceptibility, and the villain in this case was a series of exposures to moth balls. She most definitely did not have an emotionally caused tachycardia.

If this in any way seems strange to you, keep in mind this one essential fact—that moth balls are used to kill. Mothproofing is a chemical poisoning designed to interfere with the vital life processes of a special phase in the life cycle of the moth. If this chemical agent can kill moths, it is not unreasonable to think that a highly susceptible person might somehow be affected by the same toxic substance.

CASE STUDY: PULMONARY EMBOLUS AND THROMBOPHLEBITIS

Dr. William Rea, an ecologically oriented friend practicing cardiovascular surgery in Dallas, Texas, a physician with extensive experience as a thoracic (chest) and cardiovascular surgeon, states that "an ecologic orientation may alter significantly the outcome" in a variety of very serious forms of disease of the heart, blood vessels, and lungs.

The causes of both pulmonary embolus (blood clot formed in one part of the body and carried by the circulation to a lung) and thrombophlebitis (inflammation of the lining of a vein associated with the formation of a blood clot) have been an enigma. These conditions "can be very disastrous, including sudden death or prolonged disability." Dr. Rea is an expert in this field and he quotes the literature with which he is familiar indicating that diet and food allergy have been causative factors where in the past only local injury was recognized as being an identifiable cause of the inflammation in clot formation within veins. He quoted another study which reported that "a large percentage of patients with thromophlebitis were people with an allergic history."

In *Clinical Ecology,* Dr. Rea presented the case of a twenty-six-year-old woman who had severe recurrent thrombophlebitis and near fatal pulmonary emboli. The vena cava—the large vein that brings blood to the collecting chamber on the right side of the heart, from which it then goes to the right ventricle, which pumps it to the lungs—required surgical treatment because she suffered from repeated episodes of pulmonary emboli (clots to her lungs). She was given conventional treatment to prevent infection and to decrease the ability of the blood to form clots after her surgery, but she continued to have leg pains associated with swelling and redness, in addition to chest pains and shortness of breath.

After four months of constant unsuccessful treatment, she was placed on Dr. Randolph's program of comprehensive environmental control. The environment in her room was controlled in that it was as free as it could possibly be of air pollutants, and she was placed on a therapeutic fast drinking only spring water. Her withdrawal symptoms lasted for seven days which Dr. Rea described as being "very stormy." The symptoms included a psychotic episode, muscle and joint aches, fatigue, insomnia, nausea, and vomiting. At the end of seven days, she was completely free of all symptoms. The painful, swollen, and red leg had returned to normal.

She was then tested for food allergy and chemical susceptibility. She was found to be highly allergic to rice and wheat in addition to numerous chemical substances. Although she had been completely dependent on drugs that prevented blood clots (anticoagulants) for the previous six months, she was discharged from the hospital without any medication on a diet free of the foods identified by testing and, in Dr. Rea's words, "on vigorous environmental control."

At the time he wrote his report, she had been free of symptoms for eight months and was able to go to work every day, performing her secretarial duties. In 1978, I telephoned Dr. Rea and he informed me that he is still following this patient and she has remained completely well without any recurrence.

CASE STUDY: ULCERS

Ingested allergens and environmental chemicals enter the body by way of the gastrointestinal tract. After being digested, a tremendous variety of substances from the outside world pass through the membranes that line the intestines and enter the bloodstream. However, before this complex process of digestion and absorption is completed, local reactions may take place wherever these substances come into contact with the surfaces of the stomach and intestine.

Dr. Lawrence D. Dickey reported the case of Mrs. D. J., forty-eight years old, who was admitted to the hospital as an

acute surgical emergency in 1965.* On operation, a large perforated ulcer of the stomach (gastric ulcer), about three-quar-
ters of an inch in diameter, was found to be the cause of her
problem. The perforation had caused "extensive peritonitis."
(The peritonium is the membrane that lines the inner wall of
the abdominal cavity and an infection of this large surface can
be a very serious problem since enormous amounts of toxic
material can be absorbed from it. In the preantibiotic era, there
were many fatalities from peritonitis.)

Although Mrs. J. gave no history of food allergy when she
entered the hospital, Dr. Dickey eliminated milk from her
diet during the postoperative period as a precautionary measure because he was familiar with Dr. Randolph's finding
that milk allergy often was responsible for ulcers in the
upper intestinal tract. One month after her emergency surgery, Dr. Dickey tested her for milk allergy employing the
sublingual (under the tongue) technique, and she developed
acute abdominal distress, which was similar to that which
she had experienced before her stomach ulcer perforated
and led to the peritonitis. "The patient walked the hall crying and holding her abdomen." Dr. Dickey was able to completely eliminate this pain with a relieving (neutralizing)
dose of milk extract.

Soon thereafter Mrs. J. was given a series of sixteen food tests
and she reacted to three foods: milk, corn, and orange. Because
corn is present in the diet in so many forms and is very difficult
to avoid, she was given a small vial of corn extract prepared so
that one drop contained her neutralizing dose. A few weeks
later, by phone, the patient reported that her gastric distress
had recurred and persisted for several days. She was instructed
to record all that she had eaten and come to the office the next
day. The next day she appeared and stated that, after reporting
on the phone, she read the label on a can of soup she had just
eaten and discovered that it contained corn. She then took a

---

*From *Gastrointestinal and Genitourinary Tissue Eosinophils and Mast
Cells* by Lawrence D. Dickey. A Paper first presented at the American College
of Allergists Meeting in New Orleans, Louisiana, April 1967, recipient of the
Bela Schick Award. (Also appears in *Clinical Ecology*, p. 441.)

sublingual dose of her corn extract (one single drop) and within ten minutes she had relief of the gastric distress. "With the elimination of milk and the avoidance of most corn contacts and the use of sublingual corn extract as necessary, she has continued free of upper gastric distress."

CASE STUDY: ARTHRITIS

Dr. Randolph had a case of rheumatoid arthritis in a thirty-two-year-old clergyman who had suffered from intermittent abdominal cramps from age eleven to age thirty-one.* In all other respects, he had been in good health until one day he suddenly developed acute migratory arthritis involving his knees, feet, and sternum (breastbone). The arthritis was accompanied by progressively increasing fatigue and intermittent periods of mental depression.

In 1967 he was hospitalized (under Dr. Randolph's care). His left knee was markedly swollen, he walked with a limp, and the range of motion of this joint was limited to 50 percent of normal. Dr. Randolph placed him on his program of comprehensive environmental control. The patient fasted and was kept in a controlled environment. As expected, all of his symptoms got worse during the first few days in the hospital; these were typical food-withdrawal symptoms. Then his arthritis began to fade away as the effects of the causative food allergens disappeared.

When single foods were reintroduced one at a time to his diet as deliberate test feedings, the following results were obtained:

Cane sugar: In ten minutes there was stiffness of knees, dizziness, and upset stomach.

Corn meal and corn syrup: One and one half hours after this test he had stiffness of the left knee and headache, with accentuated arthritis the next morning.

Pork: In an hour and a half he became sleepy; nine hours later there was joint stiffness.

Rice: In two hours there was stomach distress, and at three hours a headache appeared.

*From "Ecologically Oriented Rheumatoid Arthritis," in *Clinical Ecology,* by Theron G. Randolph.

Wheat: At three hours there were twinges of pain followed by profuse perspiration. The next morning his left knee was swollen and painful on motion, causing him to limp.

Beet: Four hours later he developed nasal stuffiness.

After being discharged from the hospital, the patient carefully followed the diet that Dr. Randolph had worked out for him. He was also instructed to use only nonchlorinated water and to rotate his intake of foods, using organically raised foods.

It was necessary for him to eat less chemically contaminated (organically grown, natural) foods because he had arthritic and cerebral reactions to the first test meal that was given after he had finished his food tests (with organic foods) in the hospital. The test meal consisted of foods that he had tolerated during testing *but* the foods were from the commercial market and were chemically contaminated by our modern food technology. Three hours after this test meal with "regular" foods to determine susceptibility to food-related chemicals, he developed acute swelling and pain of the left knee, which increased during the night. He was unable to bear weight on his left leg the next day, and he also became tired and depressed. His knee remained painful and tender for three days; fatigue and depression continued for twenty-four hours after the contents of his intestinal tract were eliminated by the use of a laxative.

Six months after discharge from the hospital, the clergyman had a single attack of acute arthritis when he broke his diet. This convincing flareup of his symptoms suggested that he use extreme care in the future and in a seven-year follow up there has been no recurrence of arthritis. During the past two years, this patient has regained his tolerance to all of the offending cyclic food allergens that previously bothered him. His tolerance has been preserved for these foods, which are now eaten at proper, spaced intervals in his rotary diet.

CASE STUDY: EMPHYSEMA/FATIGUE/CHRONIC COUGHING

I wish to thank a very lovely lady who has kindly given me permission to use her name here. She wants people to know what we have been able to accomplish by working together.

Nadine Dorrett had a chronic cough for twenty-five years, frequent "bronchial problems," laryngitis, and "chest infections" without fever. For the year before she came to me, she had been hoarse. There were times when she "just didn't feel well at all"—and she hadn't felt really well for years. Two physicians had diagnosed her problem as emphysema, a chronic lung disease in which there is damage that leads to decreased lung ventilation with air being trapped in the lungs. As a child, every month she would be in bed to rest up for two weeks. Two weeks out of every month! Nobody knew why she had to go to bed and rest. But she really had to because her fatigue was so severe. At times she vomited, and sometimes she had heart palpitations. None of the doctors who saw her had been able to diagnose her problem. Rheumatic fever was suspected, but not seriously.

At age thirteen, several doctors said there was something wrong with her lungs, but they never were able to say exactly what the problem was. A tonsillectomy was recommended, but it was never done because every time she went to the clinic to have a preoperative examination, the palpitations would return and the doctors felt that she should not have an anesthetic. At age sixteen all of her teeth were removed because the "poisons going through her system" would kill her in seven years. (They probably suspected she had what they used to call a "focus of infection" and believed that a chronic infection of her teeth might be present and might be responsible for her being so ill for so long.)

As I took her history, the answers to her lifelong problem were there just waiting for me. Within a few minutes she informed me that she coughed after most meals and she also coughed after exposure to the fumes of a variety of chemicals. She recalled that after-shave lotion used by fellow employees and customers at the bank where she worked would immediately bring about coughing. She also related a very significant incident regarding her exposure to a toxic chemical agent that was used in her place of employment. Shortly after an exterminator came to the bank and sprayed the building, she promptly developed a very severe cough with hoarseness and distressing chest pains. In her words, "it was the worst reaction" she had ever had, but in this particular instance she was pleased that she had been able to identify the probable cause of her symptoms.

She had not taken a single social drink in the past two years because alcohol always made her extremely dizzy and her head would spin. She did, however, discover that sometimes a very small amount of whiskey would reduce her coughing (see page 36). Coffee liqueur was very helpful in stopping her cough, and the concerned and thoughtful manager of the bank where she worked kept some in his desk just for her to help control her severe coughing spasms—just a fraction of a one-ounce shot glass would usually give her prompt relief.

The weather also affected her. Dampness made her cough increase. Here we have a very probable increase in the growth of molds and an increase in the concentration of pollution factors because they are held close to the surface of the earth by the blanket of moisture. When she visited her daughter's home in Oklahoma, she coughed very little compared to the amount of coughing she did in her own home. Was there a cough-inducing environment in her home? But when it began to rain in Oklahoma, her cough increased.

She also noted that milk chocolate produced nausea and vomiting. The severity of the nausea and vomiting was directly related to the quantity of chocolate that she ate. And she would eat chocolate compulsively: Once she had a single piece of chocolate, she couldn't stop eating more of it and she'd go on a chocolate binge. (Here we have very strong clinical evidence of dose-related milk chocolate allergy and addiction.)

Her chemical sensitivity was obvious from her history. She could smell leaking natural gas before other people could. (People who are highly susceptible to various chemical substances often have the ability to smell something to which they react long before others who are unaffected by it. A very keen nose for natural gas fumes is just about a guarantee that the patient is highly sensitive.) Fresh paint fumes would cause her to cough. The odors from newly manufactured plastic articles like shower curtains, place mats, and tablecloths also caused coughing. She found that the chlorine bleach used in doing her laundry as well as chlorine-containing scouring powders made her cough. She had recently moved from a home that had gas heat and a gas stove into an all electric home, but there was no benefit from this often very helpful environmental change.

It was obvious to me that since she definitely was a chemically susceptible individual that eliminating the gas heating system and the gas stove was simply not enough. There were so many other factors affecting her, that taking the gas out of her home —even though it was the right thing to do—was only one of the many measures that were essential in a complex situation such as hers. And this is a very big problem that usually occurs in multiple allergies with multiple factors involved.

The following information was obtained by tests for foods and other types of environmental substances:

Eggs: She developed pains in her chest (which often appeared before episodes of coughing). Then she became hoarse and, finally, began to cough.

Alternaria (mold): At first she coughed moderately, but very soon the coughing became severe. She became hoarse. Her chest felt tight, and she started to bring up mucus.

Auto exhaust: She became very, very tired, and developed the familiar pains in her chest without coughing.

Apple: Again, she became tired, but this time she said she felt "woozie" (slightly confused). She coughed and developed a headache.

House dust: Her eyes became heavy and a mild headache appeared above her eyes.

Cigarette smoke: Her chest became very sore and she began to cough severely.

Milk: She yawned and yawned, and became very tired. She became very much aware of her heartbeat and said it was pounding very hard.

Chlorine: She became very tired and felt "mentally dull."

Saccharin: Her cough returned and was very severe.

Baker's yeast: There was tightness in her chest and severe coughing.

Brewer's yeast: She began coughing severely. It is interesting to note that brewer's yeast did not cause tightness in the chest as baker's yeast did, but they are different kinds of yeasts.

Natural gas: She said her stomach felt very "strange" and she developed a mild cough.

Mixed food preservatives: Usually we give three or four doses of this material, each dose being stronger than the previously given one. We had to discontinue the test after the first very weak dose, because the coughing induced by this test was quite severe and there was no need for her to have any additional exposures.

Flounder: At first she noticed a tickle in her throat. Then she began to cough moderately and finally severely. She felt very warm and began to perspire. She said that she could feel her heart pounding rapidly.

Monilia (mold): This yeastlike organism causes thrush in babies, vaginitis in women, and bowel symptoms following antibiotic treatment that kills off the normal bacteria in the intestines. She had a severe episode of coughing and a mild sensation of heaviness in her chest. She became slightly confused.

All-purpose garden spray: Her head became very foggy. She had moderate nausea, moderate shaking, and a severe cough.

House dust from Endo Laboratory: She felt extremely weak all over. She had been standing and felt she should sit down. Then she broke out in a cold sweat. She had moderate pounding of her heart and severe coughing. She said, "This type of episode happens quite frequently."

Methoxychlor: Through perseverance and the determined efforts of a chemically susceptible patient who does not, at this time, wish to be identified, we were able to obtain some of the highest quality of pure insecticides available to use for testing. The U.S. government has set standards for the exact quantity of each substance that is permitted to be taken during the course of a meal. Nadine's sensitivity to methoxychlor was so great that one millionth of the *permitted* quantity that could be taken with complete safety (according to the government) in a single meal caused her to get sharp pains over her right eye, ringing in her ears, and a lower frontal headache.

DDT: She developed a severe cough in a dose level that was about 1/2,000,000 of that permitted to be present in a single meal. DDT is no longer in use on crops, but it still persists in the soil and can still be absorbed through the root system of unsprayed crops. I have been informed that it is still used in some spraying programs for mosquito control. We know that it can be carried for considerable distances by air currents.

We started Nadine's testing on August 22, 1977. On August 25 she said she had already noticed a big improvement in her health by eating only the foods that we had determined were probably safe because my technicians had found them to be test negative. "I really notice a difference in the morning," she said, "because the morning cough is greatly reduced." On her own, she eliminated the test-positive foods and restricted her diet to the negative ones. This is an effective initial measure but she could have developed a cyclic allergy to the test-negative foods if she continued to eat them daily. Because she did have a diagnosis of emphysema from two other doctors I examined her chest, and then sent her to a chest specialist in order to obtain a set of chest X-rays. The specialist said the X-ray was definitely negative for emphysema, and diagnosed her problem as chronic bronchitis.

By November 1977, her cough was almost gone and she said, "Really, I feel great." She had lost twenty pounds, which represented some fluid retention as well as some fat she didn't need. After she lost the twenty pounds her weight stabilized.

I suggested that, like many of my patients, she follow a five-day rotary diet during which she would eat one food per meal. When we tried to add more foods, one month later, she reported that she couldn't eat two foods per meal because her coughing would start again. The net effect of two foods acting together gave her a combination she couldn't tolerate. So she will have to continue on a diet of one food per meal for a while, and we will find some combinations of foods that she can tolerate in the near future after her body has had enough time to recover from her allergic stresses.

She was not upset by being limited to one food per meal. She said, "This is the first time in my life that I have had long fingernails." And this was because she was finally free of all her nail-biting tensions due to a very reasonable concern about her chronic cough, "emphysema," and chronic fatigue.

I can definitely state from my interpretation of her past history, observations, and her responses to testing, in conjunction with her own observations and response to management based on our combined efforts, that she had unrecognized allergy affecting her lower respiratory tract for a period of twenty-five years. No one had suspected that she was suffering from a reversible disorder due to factors in her total environment that could have been identified and controlled or eliminated. I hesitate to use the word "cure," but we have accomplished a dramatic reversal in her symptoms without the use of drugs by seeking and treating the fundamental causes of her health problems. She is receiving desensitization treatment, which consists of a series of periodic injections of allergenic extracts to increase her tolerance (reduce her sensitivity) to molds and pollens. She is on a nutritional program of vitamins and minerals. And she continues to follow the diet that was prepared for her after her food testing was completed. The solution of a multiple symptom disorder which had lasted for twenty-five years was, for me, a relatively simple matter. She needed our concentrated efforts and she needed a thorough investigation. Had this been done years ago, she could have avoided many difficulties and she would have had a happier and certainly much healthier life all those years.

CASE STUDY: MOTION SICKNESS

At the conclusion of a performance at the Lincoln Center for the Performing Arts in New York, a great number of people headed for the indoor parking garage to get their cars. One woman in her late fifties was walking toward her car when suddenly she had the sensation that she was going to die. She became pale, weak, and so dizzy that she was unable to stand up. She said that the exhaust fumes from the already moving cars were "awful" and, as her symptoms increased, she had to lie down on the concrete floor. Her husband and some kind by-standers picked her up and carried her to the car, where she lay pale and exhausted.

After the husband managed to work their way out of the crowded garage he opened the car windows, and within ten minutes, she began to feel like her old self again. Then they got behind a truck on the highway leading home. She began to feel dizzy and weak again. She also noted the truck exhaust fumes and recognized these familiar symptoms as "car sickness."

Of course, in the garage at Lincoln Center, as the car engines were started, gasoline combustion products filled the air, which was already polluted with other garage fumes and tobacco smoke. Then finally she got some fresh air. She began to revive when they left the garage and opened the windows, until she got another exposure to the diesel exhaust fumes from the truck ahead of their car. She had been suffering with typical symptoms of what is traditionally called motion sickness in the garage at Lincoln Center even though she wasn't in a moving car.

As I began to put the pieces of her history together, it became obvious that she had suffered from faint feelings, weakness, occasional headaches, and dizziness almost all of her life and that this was due to the fumes of many substances derived from petroleum (petrochemicals), as well as to the combustion products of gasoline and diesel fuel.

In most of the cases of "motion sickness" I have seen, there have been very few patients who became ill from the motion of a car, train, plane, or bus. Usually, the car-associated problem had its origins in a susceptibility to petroleum-derived chemical products which are present in the car as gasoline, exhaust fumes from the engine, lubricants, and transmission fluid, and vapors given off from plastics, rubber and cements.

Dr. Harris Hosen has confirmed these findings. In his usual practical approach, he had many of his patients who had been previously diagnosed as having "motion sickness" turn their car engines on and sit on chairs that were placed in their driveways about ten feet behind their cars. Each one of these chemically susceptible patients developed their familiar "motion" or "car sickness" symptoms. Of course, there was no motion. I have asked patients to repeat Dr. Hosen's simple test on a number of occasions, and with the same results.

Allergy to the combustion products of petroleum fuels given off by cars, buses, planes, etc., can have dramatic effects. One of my patients, a ten-year-old girl, was standing at the curb where the traffic guard had the schoolchildren wait until it was safe to cross the busy street. There was a station wagon standing at the same curb with its motor running and the exhaust fumes overcame the child. She walked right into the side of the car. She was confused, disoriented, and had no concept of what she was doing until she was taken aside and away from the car exhaust.

People have been known to leave work and drive their car right by their own hometown exit on the parkway for no apparent reason. Suddenly, they seem to "wake up" and find themselves two exits farther down the road. In many cases, I believe the chemically sensitive or food-allergic drivers are disoriented and confused because they have been exposed to too many traffic fumes or their food allergy has caught up with them while driving. Their nervous systems are severely affected by their allergic reactions.

CASE STUDY: ASTHMA

Melissa L. sat facing me in my office about two years ago. The first thing I noticed was that she was rather drawn looking and had allergic shiners under her eyes (those purple-colored shadows that are the result of congestion in the blood vessels that drain the area—the slowly circulating blood accumulates carbon dioxide and becomes darker in color).

There were days when she just had to flee to the beach because it was almost impossible for her to breathe the polluted city air. She related one occasion when she awoke gasping at 3:00 AM with the feeling that someone was sitting on her chest. She rushed into the shower and turned it on as hot as she could endure and let the water beat on her face until she felt a little better. For the rest of that night she alternated between sleeping on the cool bathroom floor and on a rocking chair she wedged into the bathroom. When dawn finally arrived she leaned out the window and breathed deeply to inhale some fresh air, but she found the lining of her nose and throat hurt and burned. Trying to remain calm, she poured herself a cup of tea and listened to the morning news and weather report. The previous day's air quality had been "unsatisfactory" and there wasn't going to be any change that day. Melissa felt if she didn't get out and reach good air, she would stop breathing. She packed her bags and fled to her beach house and the fresh, clean salt air.

As we discussed her history, she told me that she always had many kinds of trouble with fumes. When she rode in a car or on a bus, she invariably became exhausted. If she spent time in the kitchen cooking over her gas stove, she could feel tension creeping across her back muscles, she would have abdominal cramping, her nose would become stuffed and her eyes itched. Her husband disconnected the gas stove when she associated some of her problems with it.

She often felt that she could breathe only very shallowly. Yet, according to a chest specialist, pulmonary function tests showed she had superior lung capacity. Then a happy accident occurred. She fell asleep late one cold night and awoke feeling quite well the next morning and realized that she didn't feel any pressure in her chest and head. Something good had happened while she was asleep. Suddenly she became aware that the room was very cool. The gas heat had stopped working during the night. She actually felt so much better, could breathe so much more easily, that she was very hesitant about calling a serviceman to repair the gas heater. But it was really too cold and damp, so reluctantly she called.

On another occasion she went shopping in town to buy an electric hot plate so she wouldn't have to use the gas stove. By the time she got to the checkout counter she was feeling very weak and thought she might faint. Barely able to keep on her feet, she paid for the electric hot plate and then ran out of the store. In the street she retched and felt dizzy, and for a moment didn't even remember why she was downtown. She felt very strange, and she added that it was not uncommon for her to feel "lost" at times when she was driving her car.

At the time she came to my office for a consultation, she was sleeping in a sleeping bag on the porch of her beach house. Whenever she had to be in the city, she slept on the top floor, to be as far away as possible from the gas heater in the basement. When she stayed at the beach house, she could breathe much better, but if a fishing troller came near the shore with its diesel engine fumes blowing in her direction, her eyes began to burn.

She knew definitely she reacted to some foods. If she ate yams, she would have abdominal pains associated with vomiting and diarrhea—but only from the yams purchased in the super-

market, not the ones from an organic food store. (According to
Dr. Theron Randolph, commercial sweet potatoes and yams are
dyed with an artificial coloring. In addition the roots of the
vegetable may be absorbing insecticides and other chemicals
present in the soil.) Spinach and eggplant gave her diarrhea;
artichokes gave her a tight chest, made her sleepy, and caused
muscle pains in her back and shoulders.

Testing at my office resulted in the following reactions:

Trichopyton (mold): She had a feeling of remoteness, separation from
   her surroundings, moderate fatigue, slight tightness of the chest,
   and hoarseness.
Hormodendrum (mold): Patient showed inability to concentrate, was
   dizzy, had moderate chills, moderate depression, throbbing in the
   temples.
Lysol: She experienced itching of chest and buttocks, tight chest and
   throat, hoarseness, confusion, was very sleepy.
House dust mites: Pressure pains in her chest, confusion, depression
   resulted.
Fusarium (mold): She became impatient, had pressure in eyes and
   lower forehead, itching of lips.
Helminthosporin (mold): These produced blurred vision, tingling of
   lips, stuffy head.
Pear: Patient had tight chest, dizziness, stabbing in the temple, rum-
   bling in the stomach.
Grape: Chest pain and blurred vision followed.
Cherry: She became feverish, disoriented, very tired, depressed.
Avocado: Negative.
Sunflower: She had sudden urge to urinate.
Tobacco smoke: She felt very itchy deep inside of her head, had a very
   stuffy head.
Tomato: She had squeezing pains in the lower side of her chest, be-
   came very depressed, very confused, very cold.
House dust: This produced waves of heat, chills, aching shoulders.
Shrimp: She had moderate tightness of the chest, moderate pains in
   her eyes, moderate sinus headache.
Yellow food coloring (coal-tar derived): She became disoriented, tired,
   depressed; felt drugged, chilly; stumbled while walking, took deep
   breaths, had a stuffy nose.

Household insects: Patient developed itching, especially in the genital area, and moderate fatigue, and then became very sleepy.

Red food coloring (coal-tar derived): She became very warm, felt a great deal of pressure in chest with severe depression, tingling of the lips; had a dull feeling in her head, a stuffy nose.

Vegetable garden spray: She developed pains in legs, generalized itching, moderate visual blurring, pain in her left knee, pain in her toes (minor arthritic symptoms).

Beef: This produced chills, moderate depression, moderate chilling, moderate dizziness, moderate occipital headache, slight hyperventilation.

Lemon: Patient had ice-cold feet, itching nose, blurred vision, inability to concentrate, moderate depression, urgent need to urinate.

Ethanol (synthetic petroleum alcohol): She had intense pressure in her temples, itching in her nose and on her upper lip. She had difficulty in concentrating. She was tired. She felt stiffness in her muscles deep inside her chest and an ache in her lower back, as though she had strained her back muscles. Ethanol is an indicator of sensitivity to chemicals, and we know she has had a great deal of exposure to plastics and gas.

Chlorine: This produced a sudden rush of heat, dullness in the back of her head. She became very tired, her head became very heavy, and she was very dizzy.

Auto exhaust: Her legs felt clumsy and weak, she had hot flashes. Her nose became ice cold and her right foot became very sleepy.

Banana: She was tired, had great fatigue, blurred vision, stuffy head, profuse sweating.

Flounder: Negative.

Weed pollen: This resulted in rush of heat, tightness in the chest, rumbling in her stomach, oppressive tightness in her chest.

Rice: She became very sleepy.

Soy: Her eyes and nose burned, she felt a rush of heat, and then she became tired, very itchy all over, developed a headache.

Almond: She had hot and cold flashes, tightness of her chest, itching, visual blurring; her stomach felt very sore; she became tired.

Lettuce: She had moderate chills, moderate frontal pressure, became very sleepy.

Melissa had been exposed to gas fumes almost her entire life. Her father's home had been gas heated, her mother's mobile home in Tucson had been gas heated. In college Melissa's dorm was gas heated. For the seven years she lived in Brooklyn Heights, her apartment was gas heated, and when she spent eighteen months in London, the house was heated with open gas fires.

She worked at a world-famous museum, making plastic dinosaur reproductions. She was exposed to plastic in the shops behind the scenes, where there is gas heating and, to compound her problems, fumes were released by the polyester resins in the dinosaur castings with which she worked.

After her diagnostic workup, I started her off on the Vitamin and Mineral Insurance Formula (developed by Dr. Roger Williams), vitamin C, and desiccated liver tablets from cattle grazed in Argentina (where they don't use insecticides, etc.) to try and replenish her body with nutrients it might need to help make her more resistant to allergies and environmental exposures. We also continued with bone meal, folic acid, calcium, and magnesium that a previous physician had recommended. I put her on a rotary diet consisting of the foods to which she didn't react or reacted to only mildly, and had her improve her environment by eliminating as many chemical exposures as possible.

Two months later she told me she was feeling better and her allergic reactions were greatly reduced in severity. She had much more energy. As a precaution against fumes from auto emissions, she had placed a special chemical air filter in her car to purify the air. Obviously she could not totally avoid coming into contact with automobile exhaust, so I prepared neutralizing doses that she could take with her and put under her tongue to stop a reaction.

On September 19, 1977, I noted on her chart that she reported she was "feeling fine" and had "no problems."

CASE STUDY: MIGRAINE/URINARY FREQUENCY/NAUSEA

One of my recent patients was an intelligent young man whose problems were thought to be completely psychological;

he was under pressure because he was a rabbi's son. For years, Richard B. had had problems with migraine headaches, urinary frequency, and nausea.

The urologists who had seen Richard suspected his urgent need to urinate many times a day was due to a virus infection of his bladder, but they couldn't find any evidence to substantiate the tentative diagnosis. For his headaches he had been seen by neurologists, who ordered skull X-rays and electroencephalograms. The examinations and tests showed nothing abnormal in his nervous system.

As part of my detective work, I asked him about his eating habits and his preferred foods. He told me that, among other things, he was eating pumpernickel bread with lettuce, tomato, and either chicken or beef very often. Pumpernickel bread is a mixture of wheat (known as the number one offender in adults), rye, caramel coloring, corn, and yeast. He also liked grapefruit juice very much and said that it made him feel "pretty good." In other words, he was getting a lift from grapefruit juice, and this meant he probably was relieving an addictive allergy to it.

I usually tell my patients on their first day of testing to be sure and knock on the door of my consultation room before they leave so that we can sit down for a few minutes and talk about their initial reactions to testing. When Richard came in with his chart we discussed the fact that he had reacted to chicken (which he ate almost every day). His reactions included headache, nausea, muscle and joint pains from which he had suffered for years. One of the very important reactions to the test with chicken was that he had to urinate four times within a half hour after the test was begun. None of the other doctors had been able to find any pus cells or albumin in his urine, and now I knew why. He did not have a urinary tract infection at all. He had an allergy to chicken which affected his lower urinary tract.

Richard had gone through a rather extensive battery of tests by the best-intentioned doctors, but to no avail. His very thorough workups had demonstrated that nothing could be found to establish a diagnosis. This case certainly suggests that if a doctor has an orientation toward bio-ecologic medicine and sees each patient as a whole entity *before* putting him in the hospital or committing him to a series of laboratory tests, a lot of time, money, effort, and possible heartache can often be saved. The fractionation of a person among the various specialists leaves a patient with an ear, nose, and throat doctor who believes that he isn't to be concerned about the current stomach, intestinal, or rectal disturbances that are occurring in his headache patient with a sinus problem. And the gastroenterologist doesn't think that he should do anything regarding the urinary tract disorder that is active while he is examining the intestinal tract (even though the urinary bladder symptoms have flared up at the same time), and they all turn to the rheumatologist because there also are muscle and joint pains. And a neurologist is called in because the ear, nose, and throat specialist couldn't diagnose this patient's headaches.

We must do away with the misconception that just because a set of X-rays do not reveal anything, or a series of blood tests are negative, and nothing is detected on examination because the involved physicians don't know the nature of the ailment, that the problem is "psychological." This young man's problem had nothing to do with the fact he was a rabbi's son and was expected to live up to a higher set of standards of behavior than any of his friends. His entire "emotionally" based health problem was food-related and I was able to prove it. He had an unrecognized multiple symptom "allergic" disorder caused by identifiable environmental factors.

Are Mental Ailments Allergic Symptoms?

If your skin, eyes, ears, nose, throat, sinuses, lungs, stomach, colon, gall bladder, joints, muscles, and heart can be sites of allergic reactions it should not surprise you that there is no reason why your brain cannot be allergic to foods, beverages (including water), molds, dust, pollens, and many chemicals. The brain is composed of living cells that were formed from the same fertilized egg as the rest of your body, and it is supplied with blood from the same kind of allergen-transporting arteries that supply all the other potentially allergic tissues in an allergic individual. Although allergic mental illness is encountered daily in every doctor's office around the world, it is rarely recognized by physicians because they don't realize allergic reactions often appear as depression, anxiety, irritability, confusion, paranoia, hyperactivity, autism, catatonia, or schizophrenia. Unfortunately, most cases of brain allergy (I call it bio-ecologic mental illness, or BEMI) are misdiagnosed as doctors search in vain for emotional causes, while allergic brain malfunctions remain unsuspected.

Case Study: Depression

One of the first cases that I recognized of BEMI was a lady who was referred to me with a sinus problem. Since she was a self-admitted ketchup freak and compulsive cravings are a sign of addictive allergy, I decided to test her for allergy to tomato, onion, cider vinegar, and sugar—some of the main ingredients of ketchup.

First I checked her with *separate* tests for onion and tomato allergy; she had moderate symptoms consisting of headache and fatigue. Then I tested her for both of these foods together by giving a mixture of onion and tomato extracts, and within three minutes she put her head down on the examining table and began to cry pathetically. Puzzled, I went over to her, gently lifted her head, and asked what was wrong, why she was so upset. "I don't know, doctor," she replied between sobs. So I asked her if there were any serious problems with her children, her husband, his job, the family finances, etc. She assured me that there was nothing in her personal life that was bothering her. Out of desperation to find some possible reason for her depression, she came up with the highly unlikely idea that perhaps she was depressed because her young daughters, in elementary school at the time, would someday grow up and leave her to get married. Of course, that explanation didn't make any sense whatsoever. Her brain was reacting to the combined allergic effects of tomato and onion, and her allergic symptom was *depression.* Depression from my mixture of some ingredients of the ketchup she craved daily!

And this patient is not alone. Over the years I have produced episodes of depression, restlessness, irrational behavior, confusion, irritability, violence, and anxiety in several thousand patients. I have also provoked severe forms of mental illness including paranoia, catatonia, schizophrenia, and manic-depression. Often, one of these unexpected mental problems would suddenly strike a patient and it would seem to come for no apparent reason—"out of the blue." However, more often than not, investigation would reveal that these problems followed a pattern. The onset of symptoms was frequently associated with many types of environmental exposures, which included foods, alcoholic beverages, water, naturally occurring airborne substances, indoor and outdoor air pollutants, drugs, and other chemical agents.

I often think about those first exciting experiences with mental illness—the lady "ketchup freak" and others with unanticipated mental symptoms that took me completely by surprise when I tested them for allergies. During that phase of my career I learned a great deal from my patients as we explored this promising area of medicine together—searching, questioning, hoping, and praying.

My initial experiences with BEMI were a major influence on the subsequent course of my professional activities. I was very excited by my early discoveries concerning the nature and frequency of cases of mental disorders due to allergic reactions that affected the brain, and through the use of simple testing techniques I was able to cause significant brain reactions in people who had not informed me that they had "emotional problems" or were currently receiving psychiatric care. Although I was testing patients to identify the probable causes of their minor physical complaints, the tests I employed were also causing ailments that were familiar to the patients but which had not been mentioned to me prior to testing. This situation occurred because none of the patients had any reason to suspect that their other symptoms had an allergic basis.

At that time, most of the patients entering the office came to me because of respiratory and skin allergies. I soon came to realize that I had to obtain a more comprehensive and a different type of past medical history from each patient in order to anticipate the wide spectrum of physical and mental symptoms that were involved in allergic responses. History-taking with new patients soon evolved into a lengthy and rather complex procedure, which became a challenging, sophisticated, and exciting intellectual adventure for me. As I gained a greater understanding from these comprehensive interviews with patients, I began to predict (to myself without telling the patients) which other allergic symptoms my testing might uncover in each patient that had not been reported by the patients when they discussed the symptoms for which they sought consultation with me. As time went by, there were many occasions in which I was able to predict these "extra" symptoms with surprising accuracy.

Since my first experiences with inhalation tests for respiratory allergy and the food and chemical tests in the case of the tomato-ketchup addict, my staff and I have performed between 300,000 and 500,000 individual tests on patients. In the process, I have proved that there is a direct causal relationship between schizophrenia and allergy in some cases of this widespread disorder. I have induced a catatonic state by allergy testing, and I have shown that many cases of childhood hyperactivity are caused by food, chemical, and inhalant allergy. In my testing rooms and in the hospital I have triggered many conditions including depression, "hysterical paralysis," anger, anxiety, fatigue, headache, learning disabilities, confusion, a sense of unreality (being spaced out), separateness, stuttering, penmanship changes, loss of concentration and memory, and inability to read with comprehension.

SALVAGING WASTED HUMAN LIVES

The first bio-ecologic mental illness program ever to be established in a mental institution was initiated in 1971 at the Fuller Memorial Sanitarium in South Attleboro, Massachusetts, after Dr. Wm. H. Philpott, the director of research at Fuller, heard about my work in the area of cerebral allergy, and invited me to the sanitarium to present my findings at a special one-man seminar. For four hours I addressed the medical staff of the hospital, local physicians, and nurses. I showed them motion pictures taken in my office that documented cerebral reactions to tests with foods, beverages, dusts, molds, animal danders, pollens, and environmental chemicals. I submitted a mass of clinical evidence that gave proof of the relationship between cerebral allergy and mental illness. I also let them listen to my tape recordings of test-induced changes in the quality of patients' voices and their manner of speaking (stuttering, stammering, and halting) and their inability to communicate ideas. Through my tapes the audience had an opportunity to "observe" the symptoms of mental confusion or depression (with crying) as reactions to symptom-duplicating tests for allergy to foods and molds and susceptibility to environmental chemicals.

After I gave this seminar at Fuller, Dr. Philpott and the hospital administrator, Mr. Gerald Shampo, asked me to accept an appointment as their staff consultant in allergy and clinical ecology. Together, we developed an excellent team from the professional staff of doctors, nurses, and auxiliary personnel associated with the sanitarium. We soon initiated a comprehensive approach to BEMI in which every patient admitted to the hospital was studied for food allergy, food addiction, susceptibility to chemicals, and inhalant allergy. Simultaneously, Dr. Philpott also conducted a comprehensive series of laboratory and psychological tests on each patient.

We showed that 90 percent of the patients who were admitted to Fuller had a significant degree of cerebral allergy. Furthermore, we were able to demonstrate that the symptoms that had made it necessary to admit these patients to a mental hospital could be duplicated by tests for allergy to foods, beverages, dust, molds, pollens, animal danders, and sensitivity to environmental chemicals!

CASE STUDY: SCHIZOPHRENIA AND CATATONIA

Because of the exceptional opportunity that was given to me to study cerebral allergy at Fuller Memorial, Jennifer R., twenty-six, is no longer a hopeless schizophrenic.* For eleven years she suffered from weakness, depression, suicidal tendencies, and episodes of catatonic rigidity.

---

*Schizophrenia has recently been reported as one of the most important diseases in this country; it requires more hospital beds than any other illness.

One of the saddest cases I have investigated, Jennifer had been hospitalized five times in other institutions before she came to our attention as an inpatient at Fuller. Over the course of her hospitalizations, she had been given all of the mind-affecting drugs that are usually employed in schizophrenia, had participated in countless futile hours of individual and group talk therapy, and had received an unsuccessful series of shock treatments. The only thing that had helped her at all was a slightly beneficial treatment with megavitamins and nutritional supplementation with minerals.*

When Dr. Philpott and I tested her for what I was later to call BEMI, we triggered a series of dramatic nervous system and bodywide symptoms as she reacted to a large number of commonly encountered substances. Our carefully selected tests reproduced all of her frequently experienced symptoms: Saccharin made her dizzy, nauseated, and anxious; chlorine, in concentrations *weaker* than in drinking water, made her depressed and afraid to swallow; lamb caused heavy sweating of her palms, mental confusion, and depression with crying. And we induced several episodes of catatonic muscular rigidity associated with its usual accompanying symptom of loss of contact with her surroundings.

As far as I know, this was the second time in medical history that the catatonic state had actually been induced in a schizophrenic patient. The first case ever to be reported in the medical literature was a patient of mine who became catatonic when I tested her with lobster extract. The test was performed after I reviewed the patient's history and learned that she had exhibited very peculiar behavior after eating a shrimp and lobster salad along with drinking a cocktail at a party. I suspected that she had an "overdose" of shellfish due to very rapid absorption when these foods were ingested with alcohol. A frame from the

---

*Dr. Philpott and I introduced Dr. Abram Hoffer (the pioneering Canadian psychiatrist who has done monumental work in megavitamin therapy) to ecologic concepts and testing techniques for determining food allergy and chemical susceptibility. About one year later, Dr. Hoffer reported that 50 percent of those cases of schizophrenia that he had not been able to help by nutritional therapy and medications had turned out to be cases of food allergy, and he was convinced that food allergy was a very important factor in schizophrenia.

motion pictures that I had taken of her as she reacted in my office was published in *Medical World News* in 1969.

Since we knew that food had been the causative factor in some episodes of Jennifer's catatonia, Dr. Philpott and I decided to find out what additional facts we could learn about her condition and determine what other benefits might be gained for this young woman if we fasted her in a controlled environment. We employed Dr. Theron G. Randolph's comprehensive technique of fasting on spring water in a controlled environment as free as possible from pollutants, and before our eyes we had the wonderful experience of seeing an unprecedented, unexpected, and miraculous recovery take place. *In four days of fasting she was completely normal!* She was no longer depressed, suicidal, miserable, exhausted, or schizophrenic.

Dr. Philpott and I continued to test Jennifer and learned a great deal more about schizophrenia in studying this very special patient of ours. We found that her nervous system was sensitive to tobacco smoke,* many molds, and house dust. Once normal, she wanted to make up for her lost years of missed living and schooling. We advised her to do so at a school where smoking was prohibited, and where there was easy access to organic foods and well water. A few months later, Jennifer left for a small religious college (where smoking was not permitted) in an area of Pennsylvania that was surrounded by organic farms. To Dr. Philpott's and my delight, not only did she complete school, but she became so well-adjusted and happy that two years after graduation we were very pleased to receive an invitation to her wedding. Within a few years we were happy to learn that she had given birth to a son.

To those readers who have lived with the anguish of schizophrenia in a loved one, I want to give hope and words of encour-

---

*In our study of more than one hundred schizophrenic patients at Fuller Memorial, Dr. Philpott and I were able to demonstrate that 75 percent of the schizophrenics had important mental symptoms from smoking cigarettes. We were amazed when 10 percent of this group of patients became psychotic when they were reexposed to tobacco smoke after they had stopped for a period of two to three weeks. *Tobacco smoke caused psychotic behavior in one out of ten!* This raised some very important questions. Should patients with mental illness smoke or be exposed to smoking? Does the smoking lounge of a mental hospital aggravate the inmates' illness and prolong their stay in the institution?

agement. There is a great deal that can be done for some patients who have this illness. At the same time, I must remind you that there is also much for us to learn about the various types of schizophrenia. Our knowledge is incomplete and we do not, and will not, succeed in every case until we learn more about this disorder.

Every patient deserves an opportunity to be well, and we must do our best to help them with the knowledge that is already at hand. Perhaps many thousands of schizophrenic patients and patients with other disorders now in mental hospitals could be helped in the same way if there were a way for bio-ecologically oriented physicians to reach them. At the present time, the doors to these psychiatric institutions are closed— along with the minds behind those doors.

Dr. Philpott and I opened many promising areas in psychiatry with our bio-ecologically oriented program at the Fuller Memorial Sanitarium. We were about to investigate many aspects of mental illness when our work was brought to a complete standstill about five years ago. We have no way of knowing what we could have accomplished in our further understanding of the causes and treatment of mental illness if we had been able to continue our studies.

The Massachusetts State Department of Mental Health prohibited our further use of allergy testing and therapeutic fasting. The Department of Mental Health would not permit us to use these invaluable methods of diagnosis and treatment in the State of Massachusetts despite the impressive supporting literature we sent to the department which indicated that several million tests had been safely conducted elsewhere and more than ten thousand patients had been safely fasted by clinical ecologists. We informed the State of Massachusetts that tests for nervous system allergy and the fasting technique had been extremely helpful in the diagnosis and treatment of patients who were fortunate enough to have been tested for cerebral allergy and to have undergone food ingestion testing after a therapeutic fast. We were informed that allergy studies should not be done in a psychiatric hospital; work of this nature was to be done only in a general hospital.

CASE STUDY: SCHIZOPHRENIA/UNPROVOKED VIOLENCE

The patient was a handsome, athletic nineteen-year-old young man who, despite psychiatric treatment, continued to have violent outbursts including physical assaults that terrorized and injured his widowed mother. In a state of desperation, Mrs. W. came to me with the hope that Michael could be helped sufficiently for him to remain at home without her living in constant fear that he would cause her severe bodily injury.

When I saw him in my office, Michael was quiet, uncommunicative, and he walked about in a heavy mental fog like a zombie as a result of the large doses of medication that were being used to control him. In the privacy of my office, as her son waited outside, Mrs. W. told me of her constant fear that he was destined for a state hospital for dangerously ill mental patients. She referred to him as "my beautiful and deeply troubled son." She could see, she said, a future that would make him a "manageable but unproductive individual" who would live a "vegetablelike existence" if I could not help him. And it was true. Michael would have been condemned to a tranquilizer/sedative-induced near vegetative existence in a state mental institution if we could not clear his mind sufficiently in order to reach him and free him.

Having been forewarned of his violent outbursts, my staff and I tested him for cerebral allergy with smaller and weaker doses of test materials than we usually employ. Each test was discontinued as soon as any irritability, restlessness, or the slightest anger was noted. My dedicated and extremely proficient technician Ester Knablin performed all of his tests with extreme care and was able to demonstrate that nervous system allergies appeared to be a major factor in the cause of his violent behavior and therefore required a thorough investigation.

Because of his volatile personality and the unpredictable outbursts of violence, it was obvious that his testing and treatment could not be completed on an outpatient basis; he was too dangerous for a comprehensive evaluation to be performed in my office. So, after discussing the problem with his mother, I made a phone call to my compassionate and wise friend Dr. David Hawkins, who is the director of the North Nassau Mental

Center and co-editor, with Dr. Linus Pauling, of the reference book *Orthomolecular Psychiatry.** Under Dr. Hawkins' care, Michael was placed in a maximum security psychiatric unit, and he was fasted for five days under careful supervision. At the end of the five-day fast, our patient was gentle and clear-thinking. Fasting stopped the harmful allergic-biochemical effects of all offending foods on his nervous system at the same time. And with this simple, safe, and inexpensive diagnostic and therapeutic measure, we were able to reach Mrs. W.'s "beautiful son," the real person inside this troubled being. His illness was reversible and there was real hope!

After he was "normal," at my suggestion Dr. Hawkins began a series of deliberate feeding tests to see exactly what role foods played in Michael's schizophrenia. Within a half hour after eating several eggs, this now pleasant, cooperative young man was transformed into a raging, uncontrollable wild animal who had to be restrained. It took five members of the psychiatric staff to prevent him from harming others and himself as he was placed in a straitjacket for several hours until his egg-provoked allergic violence subsided.

CASE STUDY: SCHIZOPHRENIA/DEPRESSION/PERSONALITY DEFECT/EMOTIONAL DISORDER

Frances C. was a twenty-six-year-old woman who stated that she had been sick most of her life. Over and over again as a child, she had been miserable, withdrawn, and unhappy, and there were periods when she would not go to school. One day she would appear to be joyful and on the very next day she would become depressed.

Although she had been examined many times, had many laboratory tests and several X-ray examinations, no unusual findings were reported by any of the doctors. Frances had been seen by a child psychiatrist and later there had been a number of admissions to different mental hospitals where a series of diagnoses were made, including depression, personality defect, emotional disorder, psychosomatic disorder, and early schizophrenia. All of her symptoms were considered to be her physi-

*San Francisco: W. H. Freeman.

cal and mental expressions of an inability to cope with her emotional problems which were supposed to be the result of some difficulties in her relationship with her mother and father. It was believed she was relieving some of her deep-seated emotional problems by unconsciously generating many symptoms in an attempt to get attention. She had been treated with numerous drugs on many occasions and had received group therapy and primal therapy.

On her first day at the office, I performed a series of tests to determine if she had an allergic sensitivity to milk, soybean, and tuna, which were among her favorite foods. Within a few hours, during the afternoon of that first day of her visit to my office, my technician had reproduced every physical and mental symptom that this patient had ever experienced! Frances could hardly believe what was happening to her; she was overjoyed. We were able to duplicate all the features of a lifetime of misery and demonstrate that commonly encountered environmental factors could bring on all of the distressing symptoms that experts had agreed were her unconscious way of seeking attention.

Although this young woman is not yet in perfect health and free from all of her physical and mental symptoms, there has been considerable improvement. She is more comfortable than she has ever been for as many years as she can remember, and this was accomplished without the use of drugs, talk therapy, or shock treatments. When she violates her diet or gets the kind of chemical exposure that many other people can tolerate, her nervous system symptoms flare up. Together, we have made a giant step toward freeing the healthy and happy person who was trapped inside a highly allergic body that was almost continuously exposed to unsuspected environmental offenders.

CASE STUDY: PSYCHOSOMATIC ILLNESS

Sandra B. was plagued by ill health throughout her infancy and childhood with "crushing" headaches and frequent episodes of acute abdominal pains. She also suffered from mental confusion and periods of depression that left her crying for hours.

Many of her doctors felt that Sandra's problems were psychosomatic, unconscious attention-getting devices. They came to this conclusion since there were no abnormal findings on physical examinations and her laboratory tests were in the normal range. When she graduated from high school, the doctors recommended that her parents send her away to college, where being on her own with her peers might help her "mature" and overcome her ever increasing assortment of ailments. College, however, proved to be disastrous for her health. On her first vacation she came home ten pounds lighter and she was, according to her mother, "the color of a shiny white refrigerator, and emotionally and physically exhausted."

During our consultation a very tired and pale Sandra B. told me that whenever she inhaled the fumes of recently applied paint, hair sprays, many perfumes, fresh newsprint, furniture polish, or floor wax she would develop a headache and become restless for a while; then she would become depressed and begin to cry. A brief period of exposure to odorous plastics such as recently manufactured shower curtains or tablecloths always made her chest feel tight and she would become short of breath and wheeze.

This information from her history was confirmed by her hydrocarbon/ethanol testing. Sandra's brain was highly susceptible ("chemically allergic") to the volatile petroleum chemicals in paint, perfumes, hair spray, newsprint, wax, and furniture polish. Her respiratory tract was very sensitive to the petrochemical fumes that gassed out from new plastics.

As we continued testing, provocation with the solution prepared from cigarette smoke caused nausea and weakness; she was overcome by a very familiar feeling that she was going to faint. (Tobacco plants are sprayed with poisonous insecticides and the dried tobacco leaf is treated with many chemicals to impart flavor and aroma; sugar is added for taste and the cigarettes are wrapped in chemically treated paper.) At college Sandra had been almost continuously exposed to the harmful effects of tobacco smoke in her dormitory, dining hall, and classrooms. These toxic fumes from burning chemically flavored and insecticide-treated tobacco nauseated her and, as a consequence, she had lost her appetite and greatly reduced her intake of food. She had suffered a weight loss of ten pounds because of inadequate nutrition resulting from a toxic suppression of her appetite.

This patient was not mentally unbalanced, nor did she have

a multitude of psychosomatic disorders which had developed because of unbearable psychic distress, "immaturity," or an unconscious need for attention-getting. She was an unfortunate victim of the unrecognized and unbearable stresses of chemical allergy. Like millions of others in our present age of chemical technology, she was susceptible to a hostile chemical environment of synthetics and pollutants for which mother nature never designed the human body to cope with.

My recommendation to this patient and her family was that she resume her academic life at another college located far from the air pollution associated with city life. There should be abundant fresh air and some nearby farms that produce organic food, and she should be in surroundings where it would be possible to avoid exposure to tobacco smoking in her school and in her residence. Sandra and her family followed my suggestions, and at college her room was turned into an "oasis" free from all chemical agents that might bother her such as air fresheners, waxes, disinfectants, polishes, etc. By a series of careful steps, she was able greatly to reduce or completely to eliminate many of the common chemical air pollutants that normally contaminate the air, and through these efforts she was able to lead a normal life for the first time.

CASE STUDY: SEVERE EMOTIONAL PROBLEMS

Vivian R., the mother of three, often became sick while doing the daily chores in her home and while shopping downtown. Within a matter of minutes after she began housecleaning or when she was in moderately heavy traffic, she would suffer abdominal cramps and have to rush to the nearest bathroom because of severe rectal urgency. In addition, her throat would become parched and her eyes would burn and itch. Once this progression of symptoms began, she would usually become dizzy and disoriented.

Extensive laboratory tests and many examinations by a number of doctors failed to reveal anything organically wrong with Mrs. R. It was concluded that she had a psychiatric disturbance, described as a "serious emotional problem." Her physician suggested that she undergo in-depth psychoanalysis after first taking a long vacation away from her husband, her children, and all household responsibilities.

The physicians who came to these conclusions meant well, but in this case, they were 100 percent wrong. They were unable to diagnose her illness because they were seriously handicapped by their total ignorance of environmentally caused cerebral and psychosomatic (brain and body) disorders. I was able to prove that her problems were not the emotional responses of a noncoping, frustrated, unhappy housewife in need of psychiatric counseling. She was suffering from what to me was a very common form of easy-to-diagnose bio-ecologic illness that could be controlled quite easily by eliminating or reducing her exposure to some important nonpersonal chemical factors in her environment.

Mrs. R. was highly susceptible to the chemical fumes from the natural gas in her kitchen stove and the odors from various cleansers and polishes; gasoline combustion products in automobile emissions also bothered her. When she cleaned her house or went downtown to do her errands, her body reacted to this man-made chemical pollution in the air, causing muscular contractions of her gastrointestinal tract, an allergic dry throat, and the very common allergic brain responses of confusion and dizziness.

I had Vivian's husband remove the gas stove with its offending fumes from their home; she eliminated all of the odorous house-cleaning products that she had been using; and I advised her to avoid the heavy exposure to traffic fumes that made her ill during rush hour and in crowded parking lots during peak shopping hours. By these measures, we were able to reduce significantly her exposure to the major environmental causes of her nervous system malfunctions. Her nonexistent "psychiatric disturbance with serious emotional problems" disappeared, and we were able to avoid the waste of time, effort, and money that would have been involved in a prolonged course of unnecessary in-depth psychoanalytic therapy.

I did what every good psychiatrist someday will be able to do. I accurately identified the nature of her cerebro-visceral allergic disorder. Then I taught this patient how to avoid the specific causes of her previously unsuspected and, therefore, unlooked-for bio-ecologic nervous system illness. This unrecognized case of chemical susceptibility would have been mismanaged by orthodox psychiatrists for months or years with talk therapy and long-term drug suppression of reactions to avoidable indoor and outdoor environmental pollutants.

CASE STUDY: NERVOUS BREAKDOWN

William V. was a young man who had been a fantastic athlete in high school, and he was generally regarded as having tremendous potential as an Olympic swimmer. For years, he won every local, regional, and state swimming meet that he entered. Suddenly, he fell to pieces and his hopes for an Olympic medal were dashed. In evaluating his problem, I soon discovered that the Mayo Clinic and a southeastern medical center were wrong in their conclusions about Bill. It was the opinion at the Mayo Clinic that he had a deep-rooted psychiatric problem involving the relationship between him and his mother. The Medical Center was certain that he had hypoglycemia.

At age eighteen, it seemed as if his productive life was over. He could barely get out of bed, he couldn't swim, he couldn't find the energy or enthusiasm to do anything at all. He was irritable, achy, depressed and exhausted. Other symptoms appeared after he entered the kitchen, where his personality would change; he would feel dizzy, light-headed, and usually developed a mild attack of bronchial asthma. A psychiatrist immediately associated the kitchen with Bill's mother and concluded that these kitchen-related symptoms revealed some hidden problem between this young man and the "dominating" personality in the kitchen—his mother. The psychiatrist felt that the underlying cause of Bill's problems originated in some repressed anger, desire, or guilt.

Because the psychiatrist was uninitiated in environmental medicine, he did not look beyond this patient's psyche. He failed to inquire about what happened to the symptoms when Bill *left* the kitchen. As I questioned him during our initial interview, I found that after an episode in the kitchen, he would always go to his room to lie down for a while, and in a few minutes he would invariably feel better.

To me, problems in the kitchen can mean kitchen chemicals and problems with a gas stove. The family was very well off and they had installed a special eight-burner gas stove in the kitchen, which I strongly suspected might be a major factor in his kitchen flare-ups. I tested Bill with Dr. Randolph's synthetic alcohol ethanol test for chemical/petroleum susceptibility and within a matter of minutes I reproduced his entire constellation of kitchen-related symptoms. And I also learned another important fact about his illness.

When his symptoms cleared, I asked Bill if he had experienced these symptoms before in any place other than the kitchen. He said, "Of course. I often get an attack of hypoglycemia in my car when I'm out driving." (Hypoglycemia is probably the most overdiagnosed condition of our day!) We talked about his sports car for a while, and I discovered that the flexible plastic or rubber mask that surrounds the base of the floor-mounted stick shift had a crack in it. Obviously, fumes from the engine (combustion products from the petroleum-derived gasoline) were seeping into the small compartment of his two-seater sports car and giving him massive overwhelming petrochemical exposure that caused the symptoms his doctors in Atlanta had misdiagnosed as hypoglycemia. Our ethanol test for chemical susceptibility reproduced his usual symptoms. Ethanol is made from petroleum, as is gasoline.

Another aspect of this case worth noting is that food addiction resulted from his doctor's treatment for the hypoglycemia that Bill did not have. The doctor told Bill that in order for him to keep his low blood sugar up to a normal level it would be necessary for him to eat foods high in protein throughout the day because protein is digested slowly and converted into liver starch (glycogen), which can provide a steady supply of blood sugar for the body. *Bio-ecologic physicians know that one should not eat the same food over and over again for days at a time. Eating in this way will probably lead to a loss of tolerance for the frequently eaten food, which will then show up as an allergic or addictive reaction.*

Bill began to eat canned chicken breasts between meals on his doctor's recommendation, and within a very short time, he started to feel even worse than he had before. He found if he didn't eat chicken every two hours, he would become dizzy, light-headed, sweaty, and nauseous—all of his symptoms were exacerbated. So he ate more and more chicken because he found that he couldn't get along without it. He had developed an addictive form of food allergy, but the hypoglycemia specialist treating him was not even aware that this possibility existed. The high protein diet overloaded his system with an excessive intake of chicken that caused addictive withdrawal symptoms —a diet-induced allergic illness. When my technician tested Bill with chicken extract (the identity of the test material was unknown to him and to me; it was just one of a series of tests being performed on him that day), she reproduced all of the symptoms for which he was eating the chicken in the first place. His well-intentioned but uninformed doctor had prescribed a dietary regime for incorrectly diagnosed nonexistent hypoglycemia that kept Bill's illness going and in fact had actually intensified it.

I was able to prove by a series of cause-and-effect tests that his breakdown was the result of a body-wide bio-ecologic illness. He had developed this illness over a long period of time because of advanced food allergy and numerous environmental chemical exposures such as swimming in chlorinated water as he trained for swim meets, exposure to natural gas fumes in his home, the gasoline combustion fumes that entered his car, years of exposure to the numerous chemicals used in the gardens around his home, insecticide residues and additives in his food, and the chlorine in his drinking water. Some of his environmental exposures had been acting on him since the time he was born, and he had had a "breakdown" when he could no longer adapt to all of the biologic stresses to which his body had been subjected.

Since money was not a factor in this situation, I felt it would be a good experience for him to go to Dr. Randolph and be fasted in a controlled environment that would eliminate all food and environmental stresses. I also told Bill to have the defective mask at the base of the gearshift in his car replaced, and I suggested that he move to the home his family had in New Hampshire so that he would be able to avoid the heavy use of insecticides that occurred in the area surrounding his Florida home. The family replaced the heating in their northern home with an electric hot-water system, which eliminated the possibility of fumes generated by burning fuel.

When he returned from Dr. Randolph's ecologic unit, he was completely well. There was only one minor health setback after that. Bill had been doing very well for several weeks and he was very happy that he had regained his health, but he wanted to be absolutely certain that it was essential for him to eat organically raised foods and continue to follow the Rotary Diversified Diet. He decided that he had to prove that "all of this diet business" was necessary, and within three days after starting his investigation with a diet of commercially raised foods and disregarding the principle of food rotation, he became weak, tired, irritable, and depressed. He returned to the diet outlined for him by Dr. Randolph, and the symptoms disappeared after he had followed his proper diet for less than five days. Needless to say, Bill was convinced. He has remained in good health to this day by following a rotary diet of organic foods and drinking spring water.

CASE STUDY: MANIC DEPRESSION/FURY/ANGER/RAGE/VIOLENCE/FATIGUE/ABDOMINAL PAIN

Wendy D., a thirty-eight-year old patient with a long history of hay fever, came to the office complaining of an irritable stomach and exhaustion. Testing revealed that her abdominal symptoms and fatigue were internal forms of pollen allergy (which were intimately related to her late spring and later summer hay fever) due to grass and weed pollens. After reviewing her dietary history and finding that she ate large amounts of beef very often, testing with beef led me to the discovery of her allergic nervous system disorder—a manic-depressive condition that she did not realize could be allergic in nature. When she was tested with beef extract, she became irritable, aggressive, and angry; then, a few minutes later, she was disconsolate and weepy—a variation of manic depression.

At my suggestion, Wendy tested herself for beef allergy at home by employing Dr. Rinkel's deliberate feeding test. This consisted of eating a large portion of beef instead of her lunch after avoiding beef for five days. Shortly after finishing the beef test meal, she became dizzy, developed a headache, became weak, and this weakness progressed to a state of total exhaustion. Finally, she fell asleep. She awoke two hours later and was amazed to find that she was in a frightening and unpredictable state of intense fury that she had experienced often in the past. These episodes of anger had never been explained. There was no relation to anything that had occurred to her which could possibly warrant such a reaction. In fact, she mentioned that she had had a very good week before she took the beef test. When she awoke from her test for beef, her entire family of innocent bystanders received the brunt of her "irrational" anger for about two hours. Gradually, her feelings of fury subsided.

Her irritability, anger, and exhaustion were very similar to the allergic tension/fatigue syndrome described in the pediatric literature and often seen at my office. It is a cut-down version of a manic-depressive psychosis. In this condition, the manic heights and the profound depression have been removed; the manic-depressive pendulum doesn't swing quite so far in either direction. The manic state is replaced by restlessness, tension, and irritability. The severe depression is replaced by fatigue, mental sluggishness, withdrawal from social activities, and easily provoked crying spells.

Wendy had not come to me because of this puzzling and frightening rage, which would erupt without warning and without provocation. She sought my assistance because of fatigue and "stomach trouble," which was characterized by belching, bloating, and intestinal gas. In searching for other causes of the fatigue and gastrointestinal disturbances, I brought about some unexpected personality and behavioral changes which she immediately recognized as being a very important and disturbing part of her life. As it had been with a number of other patients, I was able to take care of the problems that brought her to me, but I also helped her with a very serious problem that was of much greater significance to her and her family—a problem that she did not realize was even remotely connected with an underlying state of cerebro-visceral allergy. Now that she knows how to take care of herself, her life has undergone a remarkable change. She is able to work until eleven or twelve at night if she has to, and she no longer has the uncontrollable and unpredictable periods of fury that kept her family on edge for years.

My clinical experience has taught me that unprovoked aggression, hyperirritability, and different types of antisocial behavior frequently are unrecognized allergic manifestations. I know there are many marital problems among loving people, where the marriage has been or is being destroyed or where a beautiful closeness is lost, because of problems of this nature. When a person is suffering from cerebral allergy, he or she can become extremely irritable and angry either instantly or gradually. If the anger appears gradually, as the reacting person's allergic response grows in intensity, he or she will involve a spouse in situations that will almost seem to develop like a normal family argument, but there is a difference. The allergic person whose allergic symptom is irritability will pick a fight, criticize, become snippy or argumentative. Then the innocent victim of this agitated spouse, who seems to be—and really is—"looking for trouble," gets caught in the unsuspected allergic reaction trap, and both of them explode in a marital fight. Each partner is a victim in this unfortunate battle that should never have occurred in the first place. The allergic reactor was not in control and the innocent but available spouse reacted defensively to abuse or violence. I have seen several unhappy situations because of this problem. Not only is an innocent spouse the target of this fury, but the reacting spouse often feels miserable during or after the reaction. The allergic spouse may even have allergic amnesia, an allergic blackout for the entire incident. He or she won't remember what happened—no recollection of a very important event—but there may be a headache or depression or fatigue as evidence of the withdrawal phase of this recent family-disrupting reaction.

CASE STUDY: CHILD ABUSE

Other unwitting victims of bio-ecologically ill adults can be their children. A young mother came into my office and told me that she was horrified by her recent behavior. Denise R. would scream and hit her children for "nothing, nothing at all." She would discipline them for normal children's actions that needed no discipline.

Then she related a frightening experience to me. She had just taught her preschooler how to tie his shoelaces and he was very proud of his newest accomplishment. One day, as he was involved in his newfound skill, he was having a little trouble making it all come out just right, and he asked his mother to help him. But instead of patiently showing him how to do it one more time, she became incensed at his "stupidity" because he did not remember how to tie his shoe correctly after she had taken the time to teach him. She lost control of herself and in a state of anger she "slammed him and knocked him right across the room." Minutes later, Denise was sick with remorse and fear when she realized to her horror what she had done, and that she had been completely out of control.

As we worked together, testing and retesting, we discovered that she had many severe allergies that would trigger sudden allergic rage and violence. The answer to her problem was very simple. All she had to do was avoid the foods and chemicals that seriously affected her brain and she was fine. Because of my investigation, she learned if she accidentally came in contact with something to which she was allergic she could now recognize an "early warning" that an allergic attack was imminent. As soon as she noticed that she was becoming a little confused, disoriented, and her vision was blurring, she would tell the children, "Mommy is going to be sick. Mommy loves you. Mommy is going to her room to lie down." She would remain in her room until her brain-allergy-provoked fury subsided and it was safe for her to be in the presence of her children again.

MODERN PSYCHIATRY—THE WRONG DIRECTION

Initially, I had no idea how common cerebral allergy was until I began to provoke major and minor nervous system reactions almost every day, and I could hardly believe that so many people had this problem. About ten years ago, these experiences led me to the overwhelming and inescapable realization that modern psychiatry was going in the wrong direction in its search for emotional causes for symptoms that actually were unrecognized neuro-allergic responses to foods, beverages, dust, molds, pollens, and many chemicals. Because I have been able to reproduce and observe these and other mental symptoms by testing for allergies, I cannot accept the current orthodox psychiatric interpretations of mental illness which ignore the impact of environmental factors on biologically susceptible brain cells and other tissues in allergy-prone individuals.

I do not disagree with the psychiatrists who state that there are many patients who have suffered from psychic trauma or have been subjected to intense social stresses. There are many individuals in whom serious emotional damage with long-term repercussions did occur as they were growing up. A wise and compassionate psychiatrist with a comprehensive knowledge of human nature certainly can help these people whose problems have resulted from their personal interactions with members of their families, teachers, employers, or peer groups. There is a great need for clinical psychiatry that encompasses an understanding of behavioral and emotional development. It is essential that we have knowledgeable and experienced counselors who can help us because they know why we react as we do and how our emotions are affected by life's many stresses.

But beyond all this, there are many mental and emotional disorders that are allergic bio-ecologic diseases in which the biologically susceptible nervous system is malfunctioning. Most psychiatrists admit that they do not understand what a psychosis is, or what is going on in the nervous system during a catatonic state and they would fail miserably if they did not have powerful drugs and shock treatments to alter brain function. Many times all they succeed in doing is covering up the symptoms of an illness.

In bio-ecologic disorders of the nervous system, long-term hospitalization in a psychiatric facility where conventional methods are employed is often of no value whatsoever—and that means almost every hospital. Sometimes a serious form of mental disorder seems to subside spontaneously, but this is not a very common occurrence. I believe that such "spontaneous remissions" are directly related to variations in exposure to the unidentified causes of the bio-ecologic illness which waxes and wanes as the patient is intermittently exposed to substances in his total environment that reach and interact with his susceptible nervous system.

If an individual's symptoms are caused by some identifiable substances in his environment, the manifestation of this disorder can be eliminated or minimized through appropriate measures directed against the specific causes of the illness. I wish to dispense with the unproductive speculation of psychiatric theories and get down to the reality of what can actually be demonstrated in any given case of mental illness. To accomplish this, one must have an opportunity to reproduce and relieve symptoms in order to establish definite cause-and-effect relationships that correctly identify the factors responsible in each case. Those of us who investigate bio-ecologic mental illness are searching for organic causes of a nervous system dysfunction in each case that we investigate. Our goal in treatment is to correct the underlying problem. We want to eliminate the illness by identifying its causes rather than control an illness by suppressing its symptoms with drugs that merely cover up an ongoing process. We are very much aware of the fact that we do not have all of the answers yet, but we have had many successes and we know that we are looking in the right direction.

At-Home Preliminary Test for Physical and Mental Allergies

Over the past twenty-five years, my colleagues and I have found that

wheat	potatoes	chicken
corn	pork	lettuce
coffee	oranges	soy products
cane sugar	carrots	peanuts
milk	tomatoes	green beans
eggs	yeast	oats
beef	apples	chocolate

are prominent among the foods that often cause allergic reactions in our patients. This is not to say that allergy to other foods does not cause many important physical and mental symptoms.

They often do, but the above foods have become so widespread in our diet both in their usual form and combined in simple or complex mixed-food products that many individuals have become highly allergic to these foods because of their great exposure to them.

I have designed a test diet around these foods so that you can see just what physical or mental problems these foods may cause you.

THE TEST

Begin the environmental controls outlined in chapter 6. Fast or avoid all selected foods for five days before starting this test. See Appendix for detailed instructions. Then begin with Day #1.

DAY	BREAKFAST	LUNCH	DINNER*
#1	Cane sugar	Potato	Beef and *broccoli* or *cauliflower*
#2	Coffee (black)	Soy	Chicken or scallops and *melon* or *squash*
#3	Corn	Tomato and tomato juice	Pork or flounder and *cabbage* or *brussel sprouts*
#4	Egg	Milk and cottage cheese	Lamb and *lettuce*
#5	Wheat	Yeast	Shrimp or cod and *apple* or *beet*
#6	Peanut	Chocolate	Turkey or lobster tail and *carrot*
#7	Oat	Orange	Sole and *almonds* or *spinach*

*Italicized foods are optional.

AFTER THE TEST

Of course, there are only twenty-one foods* being tested on this "preliminary" diet. There are many more foods that could be causing you physical and mental problems; they must be tested too. In chapter 9, I show you how to create your own test diets (each person is unique, with unique allergies) so that you can begin to develop a list of foods to which you are presently allergic and a list of those to which you are not. Eventually, you will have tested yourself for most of the foods found on pages 241–244 until you have a group of compatible foods that don't affect you. After eating the foods that you tolerate through at least four to six rotations, retest those foods to which you reacted mildly. Some of your food allergies will be the cyclic type that rapidly lose their impact if you aren't exposed to them very often. If you do not regain tolerance after six rotations, don't be disappointed—wait and try again. Chapter 9 explains the "life style" of the Rotary Diversified Diet and how you can compensate for and adjust to food allergies so that you may not have allergic symptoms from food allergy if you don't overload your system with too frequent exposure to former food offenders.

*Excluding the optional foods.

4
Compulsive Eating and Drinking

Are You a Compulsive (Obese) Eater?

	Yes	No
•Do you feel uncomfortable if you are late for or miss a meal (headache, fatigue, weakness, depression, irritability, etc.)?		
•Do you get relief from these discomforts if you eat?		
•Is supper incomplete if you do not have a specific food with it every single night?		
•Do you go on eating binges or food jags?		
•Do you keep your favorite candy in your pocket or purse and munch on pieces of candy all day long?		
•Do you cover everything that can possibly take it with ketchup and mustard? Or relish? Or vinegar?		
•Do you have to make certain that you have a particular food or perhaps something sweet in the house all of the time? Are you afraid to run out of it?		
•Do you have trouble facing the day without a donut or two, or without some particular food or beverage in the morning?		

•Do you have to eat bread, drink milk or
coffee, or have some special food or
beverage every day for lunch or at din-
nertime or as a snack between meals
or late at night?

•Do you crave pizza, pancakes, cookies,
cake, pretzels, spaghetti, or macaroni?

•Do you have to eat a huge dish of ice cream
or something else before you go to bed
in order to sleep well?

•Do you keep a snack on your nightstand
ready for that middle-of-the-night
hunger?

•Do you insist on eating potatoes or corn in
some form at every meal?

•Do you feel there are some foods you could
not live without?

•Do you find it impossible to stick to a diet?

•Do you admit to being a "junk food
junkie"?

•Do you hide food in different places so you
can always get at it?

•Do you keep some food in your desk at
work?

•Do you still need to eat because you don't
feel right even though a diet pill has
completely eliminated your appetite?

If the answer to any of these questions is "yes," then you are
probably suffering from one of the most insidious types of food
allergy—the addictive form; and you are not alone. Millions of
men, women, and children suffer from the addictive form of
food allergy.

Unlike the better-known forms of food allergy from which
hives, coughing, itching, facial swelling, sneezing, nasal drip,
nausea, vomiting, cramps, or diarrhea result almost at once and
are telltale, readily discernible indicators that an acute allergy
is at work (and you can often make your own diagnosis), the
addictive form of allergy is much more subtle and is rarely
suspected by its victims. Why? Because instead of having an

immediate adverse reaction to the offending food, the addicted person experiences a positive feeling after eating the food to which he has an addictive allergy, just like the relief a heroin addict feels when he has another "fix" of heroin which temporarily controls his withdrawal symptoms. We do not yet fully understand why an addictive form of food allergy exists, but we know it does.

WHY PEOPLE GET FAT

Obese people are living testaments to the strength of food addiction. In a typical pattern, the compulsive eater craves and keeps eating foods with a high caloric content day after day. The foods to which he has an addictive allergy are never skipped, and eating for the relief of food-related withdrawal symptoms may become the obese person's major interest in life.

The obese person has no idea that his daily food cravings or eating habits are based on a physiologic need to stop the withdrawal symptoms caused by food addiction. All he knows is that at night he is uncomfortable until he finally yields to the need to eat the special snack he placed on the night table before retiring. This nightly ritual is followed in order to save himself a sleepy barefoot trip to the kitchen when his regular symptoms arrive right on schedule in the middle of the night. However, within a few hours after eating a food to which he is both allergic and addicted (and despite the initial good effects that may have been noted), he begins to experience familiar addictive withdrawal ("hangover") symptoms that can range from slight fatigue to severe anxiety, excruciatingly painful migraine headaches, abdominal cramps, severe depression, violent anger, panic, exhaustion, asthma, arthritis, generalized itching, and very painful muscle ache.

Progressive overweight develops as the advancing state of allergic food addiction requires increasing doses of the specific food(s) to satisfy the craving. Food at bedtime, in particular, postpones the onset of late-night or early-morning withdrawal symptoms, and eating between meals may become essential for comfort during the day. Intense, irresistible cravings make it impossible for the compulsive eater to follow a weight reduction program. He eats despite a complete loss of appetite from diet pills because food is his only treatment for the severe withdrawal symptoms that override his common sense and sincere desire to lose weight.

Eventually, the compulsive eater knows he *must* eat a certain food, to relieve or prevent mental sluggishness, irritability, fatigue, weakness, headache—his entire gamut of symptoms. A few bites of the "right" food and suddenly he is bursting with energy, his head feels fine, his personality becomes pleasant, his energy and strength return, and his thinking becomes clear again. The compulsive eater is not overwhelmed with emotional problems or an unfulfilled need for love that requires oral gratification. He is a chronic foodaholic with a serious but easily diagnosable and not too difficult to manage nonpsychological ailment.

CASE STUDY: ADDICTION TO BAKERY GOODS

Helene B., a thirty-six-year-old woman, could not "get started" for the day without having a fairly substantial intake of bakery goods. She puzzled and astonished her family by regularly eating two extra-large pieces of Danish pastry or a huge portion of pineapple upside down cake for breakfast every day.

This patient had been admitted to a local mental hospital on three occasions for episodes of depression that could not be managed in her psychiatrist's office on an outpatient basis. The last depression had been particularly severe and was responsible for her third hospital admission. Unlike her two previous admissions to the mental hospital, this time the psychiatrist was unable to control her depressed state with medications; therefore, as a last resort, he administered shock treatment.

When I tested her, I discovered she had an addictive allergy to both wheat and yeast. The allergic withdrawal state appeared every morning, causing her daily symptoms of chronic fatigue, weakness, depression, mental confusion, nervousness, headache, and abdominal pain. The wheat and yeast that she had eaten compulsively on the previous day was responsible for the appearance of her "morning sickness" the following day.

From her history I learned that she had had hay fever in her childhood during the months of May and June, the grass pollen season (cereal grains, including the wheat in her pastry and cake, are members of the grass family). In discussing her responses to alcoholic beverages, she informed me that a single drink of hard liquor (grass-family cereal grains fermented by yeast) produced many hours of extreme fatigue and sometimes caused depression during which she usually would cry for hours. I also learned that she reacted to a number of chemical fumes, including hair spray, house paint, and tobacco smoke.

I began her diagnostic studies with tests for brewer's yeast, baker's yeast, wheat, corn, malt, coffee, ethanol, and tobacco smoke. Within a few hours, I obtained a gold mine of useful information by observing her reactions to these tests—reactions that included depression, confusion, weakness, facial flushing, and abdominal pain from both yeast and wheat, and her typical gall bladder colic from coffee extract. These symptoms were easily controlled through a neutralizing process, and the wheat reaction was documented on motion picture film.

After I identified the offending factors responsible for Helene's many symptoms, it was possible to treat her in a very simple manner. Her management consisted of the avoidance of specific foods, a Rotary Diversified Diet, desensitizing injections for inhalants, and vitamin and mineral supplements. By employing the rotary diet, her addictive pattern of eating was broken and her food withdrawal symptoms were eliminated because she no longer had the food addiction problem.

This case illustrates how a bio-ecologic investigation can be invaluable in the understanding of a chronic illness characterized by monotonously recurring morning symptoms and many episodes of depression. The patient's addictive eating habits and responses to alcoholic beverages and chemical fumes, in addition to a past history of grass pollen hay fever, are recognized by bio-ecologists as diagnostic information of the greatest importance. If any of the physicians who saw Helene before I did had been aware of bio-ecologic illness, she would have been spared many years of suffering and unnecessary visits to the psychiatrist in addition to unnecessary hospitalizations, mind-affecting drugs, and shock treatments.

AT-HOME PRELIMINARY TEST FOR COMPULSIVE (OBESE) EATERS

How to Begin

The best way to approach this test is to follow the instructions in chapter 8 and fast. If you are overweight and your general health is good, fasting should not be a problem for you. On the other hand, if you have any doubt concerning your fitness to undertake a therapeutic and diagnostic fast, and if you are taking any medication, you must consult with your doctor and follow his advice.

Chapter 8 explains in detail how to go about clearing your body of food and chemical residues. But even if you are not able to fast, it is essential that you avoid all of the foods listed in the test diet for five days prior to starting your diet program. During this period of food elimination, your body will free itself of the residues of these foods, which would otherwise interfere with your test responses. If you were to continue to eat the foods that are in the test diet right up to Day #1 of your at-home test, the results would be inaccurate and you would have little to show for your efforts.

What to Watch For: Rapid Weight Loss

Many people who are obese also have noticed that their bodies are quite puffy a great deal of the time. The medical term for this condition is "edema," and it is the result of fluid retention due to an allergic response in the delicate, thin-walled capillary blood vessels present throughout the body. When the capillaries are temporarily injured during the course of an allergic reaction, body fluid passes through the capillary walls into the tissues surrounding these capillaries. Edema may be generalized or it may affect the face, hands, and feet.

After the first day or two of your fast or food-avoidance period, you may have a sudden weight loss as you eliminate this allergically retained water. I have seen a few patients lose five to ten pounds of fluid within the first twenty-four to forty-eight hours of a fast or food-avoidance period. If you suspect that you may be retaining fluids, weigh yourself twice a day while on the test diet. Weigh the food you eat each day of your diet and record the amount of water you drink (each ounce of water weighs one ounce). Check your weight loss against your intake and you will see that on some days you will have lost much more weight than the total weight of the food and water you took that day. Your big weight losses early in this program will be due to the disappearance of your allergic edema fluid.

High Blood Pressure

If you have high blood pressure and have been told to lose weight, make arrangements to have your blood pressure checked frequently or, as a number of my patients have done, you may borrow or purchase an instrument and do it yourself at home. Do not be surprised if your blood pressure is reduced and comes down into the normal range as you fast or follow the preliminary diet. Through your own efforts it may be possible to remove the word "essential" from your diagnosis of essential hypertension; you may identify specific foods that are the easily managed causes of a very common life-threatening disease.

If you do the prediet fasting, check and record your resting pulse and blood pressure at least three times a day either in a sitting or lying position after a five-minute rest period. After you start your test diet, continue to take these measurements before each test meal and fifteen, thirty, forty-five, and sixty minutes after each meal. *You may obtain vital information that could save or prolong your life. It may be possible to prevent stroke, heart failure, or kidney failure.*

Your doctor must be fully informed about your findings if there are changes in your blood pressure. Be sure to keep careful records for his information. I am certain that after he gets over his initial surprise about your good news regarding this very important aspect of your health, he will be more than happy to work out a program in which the dosage of your drug can be reduced or perhaps medications may not be needed at all. I would like to hear from you.

Test for Compulsive Eaters*

Begin the environmental controls outlined in chapter 6. Fast or avoid all selected foods for five days before starting this test. See Appendix for detailed instructions. Then begin with Day #1.

DAY	BREAKFAST	LUNCH	DINNER**
#1	**Brown rice**	**Baked potato**	Tuna or cod or **lamb** or **pork** and *squash* or *carrot*
#2	Bananas or apples and apple juice or grape juice and raisins	**Milk and cottage cheese**	Chicken or shrimp and *broccoli* or *turnip*
#3	**Puffed wheat and Matzoh and Wheatena**	**Peas or lima beans or organic peanut butter**	Sole or flounder or **lamb** or **pork** (if not eaten on Day #1) and untested vegetable from Day #1
#4	Oranges or prunes or figs or dates	**Sweet potato**	**Beef** or scallops and *asparagus* or *melon* or *pineapple*
#5	**3 tbs. cane sugar in spring water**	**Puffed corn and corn meal with corn syrup**	Turkey or eggs and *string bean* or *beet*

*Highly caloric foods are in boldface.
**Italicized foods are optional.

How to End Compulsive Eating Forever

By following the Diet for Life, Phase I, as explained in chapter 9, you should be able to lose all the weight you desire, as well as experience a level of energy and mental alertness you never thought possible. By eliminating those foods to which you are allergic—whether it's the usual, commonly known acute type of allergic reaction, or the more subtle addictive kind of allergy—

food (and eating) will assume a different degree of importance in your life. Eating will become what it was intended to be— something you do to supply the necessary fuel and building materials for your body so it can perform its natural functions, not something you compulsively have to do to stave off allergic withdrawal symptoms. Food will begin to taste good again, because you'll have the time to taste it rather than gulp it down as quickly as possible to feel better.

Cyril Connolly once wrote, "Imprisoned in every fat man is a thin one wildly signaling to be let out." Now, with your new knowledge about the addictive aspect of food allergy and a simple method for discovering those foods to which you have been reacting all these years, it is possible to release a thin and healthy person—you.

Are You a Compulsive Drinker?

	Yes	No
•Do you have to drink in the morning to start the day?		
•Do you have to drink at lunch to get through the afternoon?		
•Do you rush to the bar car on your commuter train each day?		
•Do you need to drink with supper to be comfortable for the evening?		
•Do you drink yourself into a stupor every night?		
•Do you have irritability, restlessness, headache, fatigue, depression, confusion, aches and pains, or anxiety if you miss the "happy hour"?		
•Do you feel physically or mentally better after taking a drink?		
•Do you have insomnia if you don't drink before bedtime?		
•Do you have hangovers?		

•Does the "hair of the dog that bit you" make you feel better?

•Do you have alcoholic blackouts with no recollection or memory of recent events that occurred during a few hours, an evening, or a period of several days?

•Do you have an inability to stay "on the wagon"?

•Do you stop your housework for a drink during the day?

•Do you keep alcohol in your desk for a quick one at work?

If your answer to any of these questions is "yes," it is highly probable that you are showing the signs and symptoms of what Dr. Theron G. Randolph calls the acme of food allergy—an addiction to alcoholized foods—alcoholism.

COMPULSIVE DRINKING IS RARELY PSYCHOLOGICAL

After Dr. Rinkel and Dr. Randolph discovered and enlarged their understanding of the addictive form of food allergy, a whole new perspective on compulsive drinking emerged. Dr. Randolph realized that in many cases compulsive drinking is a form of food addiction, and alcoholism an addictive physical disorder, not a psychological or emotional problem.* An alcoholic may think (or have been told) that he is drinking to combat an anxious or depressed state of mind due to some emotional problem—and a drink certainly makes him feel better fast— but, in reality, he is suffering from the addictive form of food allergy, and his anxiety and depression are nervous system allergic reactions to the food residues of the source materials in the alcoholic beverage.

Alcoholic beverages are derived from the fermentation of

*Dr. Randolph described compulsive drinking as an addictive disorder in a comprehensive paper published in the *Quarterly Review of Alcoholism* in 1956.

sugars derived from the plant starches of a variety of grains and vegetables or are naturally present in fruits. Bourbon, for example, is distilled from the fermentation product of corn, barley (malt), rye, and yeast. Domestic vodka contains corn, barley (malt), rye, wheat, potato, and yeast, and possibly beet sugar and cane syrup. Beer contains corn and barley malt; grape is in wine; cane is in rum. They all contain brewer's yeast.

The presence of alcohol accelerates the absorption of materials from the upper intestinal tract into the system. As alcohol is absorbed, it carries along with it the specific foods from which that particular alcoholic beverage was derived (as well as foods or drugs ingested along with the alcohol). Any and all of the ingredients from which alcoholic beverages are made can produce an "addictive" form of advanced food allergy in a person who then becomes a compulsive drinker. Like the compulsive eater, the compulsive drinker suffers from withdrawal symptoms from one or more of the food ingredients in his favorite drink. These alcohol-related withdrawal symptoms often are so intense that the addicted drinker is driven to seek relief from his discomfort by having another drink, and the cycle goes on and on.

As Dr. Randolph described it, compulsive drinking is the alcoholic's way of postponing hangovers by taking more alcohol as soon as the hangover symptoms appear. Unfortunately, as in any addiction, more frequent and larger doses are very often needed to control withdrawal symptoms and briefly regain the feeling of well-being. In cases of compulsive drinking, there is a vicious cycle of withdrawal symptoms and relief which is followed by recurring symptoms that are temporarily relieved by the ingestion of still more alcohol until this endless cycle is permanently interrupted.

In a recent radio discussion on alcoholism, the physician guest speaker indicated that a substantial number of alcoholics were chronically ill young adults who took their first drink while they were in their teens and found they loved alcohol instantly because it made them feel so much better. The doctor presented this fact, but he did not recognize its significance. To one who understands the addictive aspect of food allergy, it is easy to understand why these young people became compulsive drinkers so quickly. For many years they had been suffering from the effects of chronic addictive food allergy.

A young person could have been ill for years because of addictive wheat allergy that was perpetuated by eating bread, cake, cookies, pretzels, crackers, pizza, and spaghetti. Then, as if by magic, his chronic symptoms were almost instantly relieved when he took his first drink of a wheat-derived alcoholic beverage. That first very special drink "cured" symptoms that had been present for many years because the rapidly absorbed alcoholized wheat blocked the effects of the food withdrawal that were making him ill. The first drink was thus the beginning of a downward spiral into an increased intake of alcoholic beverages which were rapidly effective food addiction treatments via rapidly absorbed food alcohol.

HOW A COMPULSIVE DRINKER CAN HELP HIMSELF

The compulsive drinker is suffering from an addictive form of food allergy to one or more of the foods employed in the production of his favorite drink. The addicting foods are usually present in his daily diet. For him to be cured, we must identify the particular food allergens in his compulsively taken "favorite" drink and eliminate these foods from his diet completely or he will keep craving the alcohol that contains them.

In fact, without a single test, a compulsive drinker could conceivably eliminate all of the alcohol source foods from his diet by finding out the ingredients of his craved alcoholic beverage(s) and make very satisfactory progress in controlling problem drinking. As long ago as 1948 Dr. Randolph was the outstanding investigator involved in allergy-oriented studies of alcoholism. I am indebted to Dr. Randolph for supplying me with the following case history of an abstaining alcoholic who had not had any form of alcoholic beverage for twenty-six months when he first came to my colleague. Dr. Randolph put him on a special diet that eliminated malt, wheat, rye—the major ingredients in the patient's favorite drink. For three days this reformed compulsive drinker, even though he had not had a drink in twenty-six months, went through a period of incapacitating withdrawal symptoms. Two days after these symptoms cleared up, he had a test meal consisting of wheat only, and this cereal grain triggered a "hangover" that was, according to the patient, indistinguishable from the morning-after syndromes that he had associated with his past drinking.

Obviously it was not the ethyl alcohol present in these beverages that had been at the root of his drinking problem—it was an addictive food allergy to the wheat from which the alcohol was derived. (As you can see, the words "hangover" and "withdrawal" are interchangeable.) He had abstained from drinking, but not from the foods that were the source of his drinks. He had maintained the same old wheat addiction, but he fought it on a different level by getting his daily wheat "fix" for twenty-six months by eating foods that contained wheat and this held his wheat symptoms in check by preventing his withdrawal hangovers until he stopped eating wheat.

Thanks to Dr. Randolph, we have known about the addictive aspect of food allergy and its role in alcoholism for decades now, but this valuable information has fallen on deaf ears. I believe that most of the profitable sanitariums for alcoholics could be closed up permanently if we had an opportunity to employ the available bio-ecologic techniques, including appropriate nutritional therapy, in some institution where we could observe, control, and cure such patients.

CASE STUDY: ADDICTED TO SWEETS AND ALCOHOL

One of my patients, Rebecca S., a forty-nine-year-old nurse, was very concerned because she believed she was suffering from a serious ailment that no one could diagnose. She had been "going downhill for two years" with constant fatigue, nausea, and headaches. She was certain the doctors were not telling her the truth about how bad things really were.

She gave a history of chronic nasal symptoms and moderately severe earaches that began in early childhood and continued to bother her throughout her adult years. She also suffered from insomnia and regularly awoke at 3:00 AM feeling very restless. There were occasional lapses of memory with frightening and embarrassing periods of confusion. (During conversations there were times when Rebecca would be unable to complete a sentence, and there were a number of occasions when she unexpectedly found herself stuttering.) She also suffered from pains in her leg and thigh muscles, and often experienced pain and stiffness in several of her joints.

Alcoholic beverages had a profound effect on her. She usually became stuporous after drinking a single bottle of beer. Yet Rebecca had an intense craving for beer every night because she found it impossible to fall asleep without it. One cocktail would regularly produce a very frightening reaction. "Manhattans and martinis are disasters for me!" she told me. Within two to four minutes she would become "numb all over" and find it difficult to move. At its worst, her reaction to cocktails made her so weak that it was necessary for people to help her to her feet. Once up, she would be extremely light-headed and stagger as she walked. The next day she would always be lethargic and achy, and would feel detached and alone as if she were not really in contact with her surroundings. And, of course, she would awake with a severe hangover, which is characteristic of addictive allergy.

In addition to this enlightening information regarding the immediate and delayed effects caused by alcoholic beverages, she also told me that she was affected by tea, chocolate, and "sweets." She had an irresistible need to eat a chocolate bar every evening, to drink tea throughout the day ("I always have a cup in my hand"), and she frequently craved bakery goods such as pies, cake, and cookies.

I began her food tests with the above information from her personal observations to guide me, and I suspected that tea and some of the ingredients of those incapacitating cocktails, beer, chocolate bars, and bakery goods were probably major allergic offenders. My initial diagnostic impression, which was based entirely on her excellent history, was confirmed during her first testing session in my laboratory. Her reactions to tea, chocolate, bakery products (yeast), and alcoholic beverages (yeast and corn) reproduced *all* of her complaints. I instructed her to eliminate these food offenders from her diet immediately, and within a week she had a remarkable improvement. All her symptoms disappeared and she no longer craved chocolate, beer, bakery goods, or tea; because this one-week period of food elimination was all that was required to break the food addiction that had made her ill for years.

In this case, the solution to a serious problem was a very simple matter which required only a few office visits. We cannot always succeed like this with every patient who seeks our assistance, but there are so many people who could be so much better. They must have an opportunity to benefit from bioecologic methods of diagnosis and treatment, and we must see to it that this information reaches every physician.

CASE STUDY: COMPULSIVE DRINKING IN A SEVENTEEN-YEAR-OLD BOY

A young man, age seventeen, who seemed to be very bright and have great potential, came to my office recently with the complaint that there were days when he was just too tired to get up, or if he could manage to get up, he would be unable to do well in school. His family often found him drunk, and they were much concerned that he might be afflicted with "genetic alcoholism," because there were a number of alcoholics in the family.

This young man told me that he really loved beer, and it was impossible for him to resist it. He also loved creamed corn. (Remember, almost every brand of beer is made by the brewer's yeast fermentation of corn sugar—glucose (dextrose) —that is derived from corn starch.) When I tested him I found that he was allergic to all of the components of creamed corn. The corn made him slightly depressed and tired, the milk in the cream sauce made him slightly tired, and wheat in the flour in the cream sauce caused him to become exhausted. The most dramatic reaction of all in this beer lover, however, was the one I produced when I tested him with brewer's yeast. He was unable to remain awake, and it was necessary for us to assist him from the testing room and have him lie down on a couch where he slept soundly for half an hour. A few minutes after he awoke, he telephoned his mother at home, but he was in such a confused mental state and his voice was so altered that his mother did not recognize his voice, and she thought that she was the

victim of a crank call. "But I'm your son," her son kept insisting
—only he could not remember his name. Finally, he said,
"Mother I'm the one that works in the garage!" and then she
realized who it was, but, because of the change in his voice and
his confusion due to the test with brewer's yeast, she was certain
that her son was drunk. The yeast reaction was indistinguishable from his all-too-frequent episodes of intoxication from beer.
The combined effect of his sensitivity to all of the beer source
materials had to be a terrible biologic stress.

Was his compulsive drinking hereditary? He probably did
inherit the capacity to get into this trouble because he most
likely was born with some hereditary enzyme deficiency that
made him biologically incapable of handling corn and brewer's
yeast. I believe that some of these inborn deficiency states are
really metabolic errors that can be improved or controlled by
appropriate meganutrient treatment, and this aspect is being
investigated by men like Dr. Roger J. Williams (see chapter 7
on nutrition).

Present management in this case consists of a desensitizing
program to dust and molds (some respiratory and cerebral
symptoms were provoked when he was tested for dust and
mold sensitivity), an elimination diet that avoids all foods to
which he is allergic, a nutritional program with multivitamins
and minerals, large doses of vitamin C, and organic desiccated
liver in dye-free capsules.

ALCOHOLICS ANONYMOUS

AA has the best of intentions, but unfortunately it is often
attempting to deal with compulsive drinking that is actually an
advanced form of addictive food allergy. No amount of the
"buddy" system or calling upon a "higher power" is capable of
eliminating food addiction. The compulsive drinker, and I can't
emphasize this point too strongly, *must* find out if addictive
food allergy is the cause of his problem with alcohol. Because
if it is, and he gives up the alcoholic beverages that contain the
foods to which he is addicted but does not eliminate those same
foods from his diet, he is never going to be free from the symp-

toms that he is able to *relieve* temporarily by drinking in the first place.

I attended five local AA meetings as a guest observer several years ago to learn about their program because some of my patients were heavy drinkers. During a period following one of the meetings, I raised the issue of food allergies and asked if anyone attending the meeting was aware that he might have them. A number of hands shot up, and some of the members said that they also had allergic reactions to alcohol. However, no one had ever told these people that if they were allergic to commonly eaten foods such as wheat, malt, barley, sugar, corn, rye, yeast, etc., which are the ingredients present in alcoholic beverages, that there would be a delayed allergic addictive reaction triggered by these foods when they drank alcoholic beverages prepared from them, as well as when they ate them.

The directors of AA have been made aware of these facts, but they resist this knowledge about food addiction as a major cause of compulsive drinking because it doesn't fit into alcoholism as they see alcoholism. They do claim some "cures." Yet, according to Dr. Randolph, the "successes" of AA are quite limited and actually may happen only when the compulsive drinker finds that the drink that used to give him relief no longer does so and now makes him ill.

AA literature states that *you* can't help the alcoholic, only he can help himself, but without knowledge this is not possible in the case of addictive drinking. AA says the alcoholic has to hit a "rock bottom," but this rock bottom state is not when he has lost his job, house, car, wife, and children. *It is when his body's adaptation mechanism fails and the alcoholic has lost his ability to tolerate any alcoholic beverage and he must stop drinking because the symptoms from drinking make him feel worse than abstaining.* He used to have nausea, now he actually vomits. He used to get headaches, now he has severe migraines. He used to tremble, now he shakes violently.

A message I once saw scrawled on the wall of a restaurant men's room read, "Death is Mother Nature's way of telling us to slow down." The "reformed" alcoholic has heeded a similar message, but that kind of "cure" takes a long, long time.

The allergic alcoholics who are able to stop drinking before their adaptation mechanism fails are those individuals who get relief from their withdrawal symptoms by eating the foods to which they are allergic and addicted. Instead of drinking rapidly absorbed alcoholized foods for relief, many abstaining "reformed" alcoholics have an instantly available pocketful of corn, malt, and sugar-containing candy or raisins, or they may compulsively drink sugar-sweetened carbonated beverages (soda pop) or eat wheat, corn, oats, barley (malt), or rye-containing food products in a manner that relieves or blocks withdrawal symptoms.

Although AA and its related organizations have only the best intentions, they often fail just like many of the sincere physicians, psychologists, and social workers who have tried to cure compulsive drinkers. Counseling, psychoanalysis, group therapy, family therapy, and medications cannot help the compulsive drinker get to the biologic root of his problem if his alcoholism is an addictive form of food allergy that is never recognized or properly treated.

AT-HOME PRELIMINARY TESTS FOR COMPULSIVE DRINKERS

Because each compulsive drinker may have a "favorite" drink, I have divided the at-home tests into four categories for simplicity's sake:

1. Grape wine drinkers' test
2. Beer drinkers' test
3. Rum drinkers' test
4. Whiskey drinkers' and vodka drinkers' test

All alcoholic drinks have certain ingredients in common. Individual kinds have a few ingredients unique to that particular beverage. In each test diet, the commonly found food ingredients in a specific drink are in boldface. You may be allergic or addicted to foods common to several alcoholic beverages (yeast, corn, malt, etc.) or to some food ingredients that are found only in a specific drink. Note that there are other foods you will test yourself with that are not found in alcoholic beverages, but these foods may also cause allergic difficulties.

If your favorite drink is a mixed drink like a screwdriver, which contains orange juice, a Bloody Mary made with tomato juice, or a Tom Collins containing grapefruit juice, you could be allergic to these rapidly absorbed juices as well as to the ingredients employed in the production of a specific type of alcoholic beverage. If your particular mixer does not appear on the diets in this chapter, you will have to test it later in the Diet for Life, Phase I (chapter 9).

Many compulsive drinkers unfortunately reach a state where they are unable to keep a job and they can easily perform these tests at home. If the compulsive drinker is working, he probably is performing at only a fraction of his capacity, and he owes it to himself, his family and his employer to take a brief period of sick leave to work out this serious problem. If he feels he cannot adhere strictly to the test diet while working, he must take time off to conduct these tests at home.

How to Begin

The best way to approach any food test, is to fast for five days prior to the testing (see chapter 8 and Appendix). If you feel that you are unable to fast for whatever reason, you must eliminate alcoholic beverages and every food listed on your specific alcoholic test from your diet for five days prior to beginning the test. If you continue to include these foods in any form whatsoever in your diet, you will not be able to interpret your reactions correctly. You must give your body time to free itself of any food residues from the foods that will be used in your tests so that you can have an unmasked acute reaction to them. It is a complete waste of time and effort if you continue to eat them or to drink right up to Day #1 of the diet. This is your chance to find out if you are suffering from an addictive form of food allergy—whether your drinking habit may possibly be the result of a nutritional disorder. There is a slight chance that it may represent a psychological problem. Do it right. It is *your* life. The results can very well be worth the effort.

Discussion

Diet testing for the individual food components of alcoholic beverages will seem to be a rather simple procedure at first glance. Do not be misled by the apparent simplicity of this test because you cannot obtain accurate results unless you follow my instructions very carefully. If you react to any food test, do not eat your next test meal until all symptoms are gone. If you have to omit a feeding because of a reaction, you will have learned something very important and it is very much worth your while to postpone eating and take whatever additional time is necessary for you to complete this at-home test—it may provide information that is helpful to you for the rest of your life.

It is possible that you may have unrecognized (masked) allergy to some of the foods that you will eat during this test. You may be quite surprised to find that you react to foods that you have never suspected were affecting your health. One of the major problems involves "hidden" foods which may be present in various food mixtures and are very difficult to avoid unless one takes special care to do so. Milk, wheat, eggs, corn, sugar, yeast, and soy are prominent among the hidden foods, since they frequently are components of many food products. Your difficulty is increased by the fact that there are many standardized food mixtures that we recognize by a name such as ketchup or milk chocolate. Only the name of the product need be stated on the label since the manufacturer must comply with government standards for the manufacture of this particular food. There are many ingredients in a bar of milk chocolate in addition to the milk and the chocolate—at least fifteen substances may be present. With respect to ketchup, the government requires that a certain amount of tomato be present, but there are several types of vinegar or sugar that may be used and these allergically significant components can vary from brand to brand and from time to time in the same brand. For example, ketchup may be sweetened with either corn sugar, cane sugar, or beet sugar. There is no way for a consumer to tell the kind of sugar that is present in the bottle of ketchup he purchases. Even if he continues to use the same brand exclusively, he can never be certain regarding this matter because the manufacturer's selection of a sweetening agent is based upon available supplies and the current price of each type of sugar.

In the five-day period in which you are preparing to follow this diet, it is quite possible that you will have difficulty in avoiding corn. Your first reaction to this statement may be, "If

I don't eat ears of corn or canned corn, and I stay away from corn relish and corn flakes, corn should not be a problem for me." Unfortunately, this is not the case because corn is one of our most widely used food substances, and it is very difficult to avoid in the form of corn sugar, corn syrup, cornstarch, and corn oil.

Warning: If you have ever been hospitalized for or experienced alcoholic delirium tremens (DTs), *do not take this test* without being under the very close supervision of a physician. Withdrawal symptoms can be dangerous in your case, and testing with the foods found in your "favorite" drink may make you moderately or severely ill because allergic symptoms to these foods often are exaggerated by this technique.

Test for Grape Wine Drinkers*

Begin the environmental controls outlined in chapter 6. Fast or avoid all selected foods for five days before starting this test. See Appendix for detailed instructions. Then begin with Day #1.

DAY	BREAKFAST	LUNCH	DINNER**
#1	Orange, grapefruit, or pineapple juice (2 glasses)	Apple or tomato juice (2 glasses)	Lamb, scallops, or cod and *carrot*
#2	Banana or melon	Sweet or white potato	Shrimp or chicken and *peas*
#3	Pear, dried figs, or prunes	**Raisins or grapes** and grape juice (2 glasses)	Beef† (or any of the Day #1 or Day #2 dinner foods except cod) and *broccoli*
#4	Strawberries, peaches, or another type of melon	**Beets and 2 tbs. of beet sugar** in spring water	Sole or flounder (or food from Day #1 or Day #2 dinner that you have not yet had) and *string beans*
#5	Milk (2 glasses) and cottage cheese	**Brewer's yeast**—2 tbs. in one of the juices from Day #1 breakfast or lunch	Pork or turkey and *cabbage* or *turnip*
#6	**Cane sugar**—3 tbs. in a glass of spring	**Corn** meal mush with corn syrup	**Eggs‡** (or any dinner food from Day #1

water

that you have not
tested if you can't
eat eggs), *lima
bean* or *squash*

*Foods found in grape wine are in boldface.
**Italicized foods are optional.
†If not eaten on Day #1 or Day #2.
‡Used in clearing some wines.

Test for Beer Drinkers*

Begin the environmental controls outlined in chapter 6. Fast
or avoid all selected foods for five days before starting this test.
See Appendix for detailed instructions. Then begin with Day
#1.

DAY	BREAKFAST	LUNCH	DINNER**
#1	Pineapple, grapefruit, or orange juice	Tomato or apple juice	Turkey or pork and *squash* or *pumpkin*
#2	Bananas or prunes	**Brown rice**	Lamb or scallops and *cabbage* or *broccoli*
#3	Grape juice and raisins or pears	Sweet potato or peas	Cod, haddock, or chicken and *carrot* or *celery*
#4	**Barley and malt**	Baked potato	Beef, crab, or shrimp and *lettuce* or *pecans*
#5	Melon or strawberries	**Brewer's yeast in juice from Day #1**	Halibut, sole, flounder, or eggs and *nuts*
#6	**Corn meal mush with corn syrup (Karo)**	Milk and cottage cheese	Pork,† lobster tail, or lamb and *lima* or *string beans*

*Foods found in beer are in boldface.
**Italicized foods are optional.
†If not eaten on Day #1.

Test for Rum Drinkers*

Begin the environmental controls outlined in chapter 6. Fast or avoid all selected foods for five days before starting this test. See Appendix for detailed instructions. Then begin with Day #1.

DAY	BREAKFAST	LUNCH	DINNER**
#1	Orange, grapefruit, or pineapple juice	Tomato or apple juice	Lamb, shrimp, or scallops and *squash*
#2	Banana or strawberry or peach	Peas, sweet potatoes, or broccoli	Chicken, haddock, or cod and *lettuce*
#3	Oatmeal or barley or pear	Cottage cheese and milk	Beef, crab, or lobster tail and *baked potato*
#4	Melon, prunes, or apricot	Grape juice and raisins	Turkey or eggs and *beets* or *cabbage*
#5	**Cane sugar**—3 tbs. —in spring water	**Brewer's yeast**—2 tbs. in juice from Day #1	Pork, sole, or flounder and *turnip* or *lima beans*

*Foods found in Jamaican and domestic rums are in boldface. Jamaican rum is grape-free.
**Italicized foods are optional.

Test for Whiskey and Vodka Drinkers*

More time is needed to work out this complex and most serious problem since many foods are employed in the production of these alcoholic beverages. Cereal grains must be taken on alternate days in order to obtain clear-cut results. This test diet requires more time than the others, but your health, family life, and job may be in grave danger and you must follow these instructions to help yourself as much as possible.

Begin the environmental control, outlined in chapter 6. Fast or avoid all selected foods for five days before starting this test. See Appendix for detailed instructions. Then begin with Day #1.

DAY	BREAKFAST	LUNCH	DINNER**
#1	Orange or grapefruit	Oatmeal	Chicken or shrimp and *broccoli* or *turnip*
#2	Apple or pineapple	**White potato**	Pork, sole, or flounder and *peas* or *lima beans*
#3	Bananas, strawberries, or prunes	**Rye** (cereal or crackers)	Turkey or lobster tail and *carrots* or *raw cashew nuts*
#4	Melon or pears	Beets and beet sugar	Lamb or scallops and *lettuce* or *asparagus*
#5	**Corn meal mush and corn syrup (Karo)**	Repeat corn test	Cod or haddock and *sweet potato*
#6	Uneaten fruit from Day #1	**Yeast**	Uneaten selection from Day #1
#7	**Wheat (Matzohs) and wheatena**	Repeat wheat	Egg, tuna, or salmon and *cabbage* or *spinach*
#8	Uneaten fruit from Day #2	**White potato**	Uneaten selection from Day #2
#9	**Barley**	—	—

*Major foods found in straight and blended whiskey and vodka are in boldface.
 **Italicized foods are optional.

THE CURE OF THE FUTURE

Bio-ecologists know if you are reacting to something you have eaten or to a testing solution, eating a very, very small amount of that same reaction-causing food or receiving a weak dose of the test material by injection or as under-the-tongue drops will often stop the reaction. While I was working as a consultant in allergy and ecologic diseases at the Fuller Memorial Hospital with Dr. William Philpott, I decided to try this neutralizing technique as a possible method of controlling compulsive drinking in some of our alcoholic patients. I had already relieved active hangovers with it in my office, and I had provoked typical hangover symptoms in an abstaining alcoholic by giving him food tests.

One of the alcoholic patients was a young woman, a teacher, who had been drinking a quart of wine each day for several years. We purchased a bottle of the wine she had been drinking compulsively, and I made a series of dilutions from this beverage in distilled water and tested her with various concentrations. This is the first time in medical history that alcoholics were treated with dilutions of the alcoholic beverages to which they were addicted and drinking compulsively. It was a carefully done trial-and-error procedure as I hopefully sought to find the "hair of the back of the dog" neutralizing dose that I theorized would stop her addictive craving for wine. After several attempts, I finally did find the treatment dose I was seeking —0.1 cc of wine and 1000 cc of water, which is equal to about two drops of wine in a quart of water.

Once I had determined the correct neutralizing dose of highly diluted wine that completely eliminated her addictive craving for this alcoholic beverage by relieving her withdrawal symptoms, it was a very simple matter to mix up a batch of anti-wine treatment material for her. Instead of drinking the large amounts of wine that she formerly took when she had an uncontrollable urge to drink, she needed only to take teaspoon doses of her neutralizing solution. In less than three weeks it was possible to wean her—painlessly, without DTs—from the alcoholic beverage that had dominated her life for several years.

Just think of it. One teaspoon of highly diluted wine containing about 1/2000 of a cc of wine could be taken several times a day and it controlled her alcoholism completely. A few teaspoons of extremely diluted wine completely replaced her former daily intake of one quart of wine. If she required as many as 10 teaspoons of this neutralizing solution per day, this would be equal to substituting 1/200,000 of a quart of wine each day for an entire quart. Carrying these figures out to their ultimate, I calculated that the amount of treatment material that could be prepared from one quart of wine would last her 548 years if she were to need it daily. Her alcoholism, if it were to persist at its present level, would be controlled at a cost of one to three cents per year under present economic conditions.

Another alcoholic patient, a neighbor of mine in his middle years, began each drinking day in the same way. He started every morning with 1½ ounces of blended whiskey, which he mixed with 3 ounces of milk. Every day between 8:30 AM and 3:00 PM he took from five to six drinks of this whiskey and milk mixture. If he did not have this food and alcohol combination by 9:00 AM every day, his speech would become slurred, he would feel physically and mentally sluggish, and his scalp would itch severely, causing him to scratch himself frantically. (He had linear scars and scabs on the balding area above his forehead as a consequence of his frequent scratching during his regular morning withdrawal period.)

Since his craving for this drink began at 8:30 in the morning, I told him to come to the office on a Sunday morning at 8:30. He did and, as requested, he brought me an ounce of his favorite whiskey to make treatment material from. I did not allow him to take his scheduled 8:30 AM drink, and I watched him carefully, noting instead the progression of his withdrawal symptoms. By 10:00 AM he was so fatigued that he could hardly keep his eyes open; his speech was slurred and he sat in front of me scratching his scalp. Then he became agitated and said that he really had to have his regular whiskey and milk. He needed this drink quite badly, and he did not think he could wait any longer for it.

By this time, I had prepared a series of dilutions of his blended whisky with the hope that I would be able to find a neutralizing dose with which I could relieve his addictive withdrawal symptoms and thereby control his need to drink. The first dose I selected was not the correct one and his symptoms immediately become worse. I tried another dose of the diluted whiskey, and the result was prompt and dramatic—all of his symptoms cleared. Leaning back in his chair and with an amazed expression on his face, he said that the treatment made him feel "so tranquil" he hadn't felt that good in years.

He had absolutely no desire to drink! A small fraction of a single drop of his favorite drink did the trick—but it had to be just the right amount. The beneficial effect of this minute neutralizing dose lasted for three full days, during which he was completely free of any desire to drink at all. As with the wine-addicted alcoholic schoolteacher, his symptoms were also controlled by a tiny fraction of the alcoholic beverage to which he was addicted and which he was drinking compulsively. This single neutralizing dose eliminated his need for between fifteen and eighteen glasses of his milk and whiskey mixture a day. Less than one drop of the alcoholic beverage was able to replace an intake of about one and one-half pints of whiskey and control his compulsive drinking.

My big regret is that I was not able to study him for any length of time, nor to determine whether he also had a milk problem. Shortly after our highly productive initial visit, he was transferred to another city.

I have extended the clinical application of Carleton Lee's neutralizing treatment. The treatment I have developed and given to a limited number of compulsive drinkers has shed a new light on a very promising approach that should influence the future course of treatment in alcoholism. Although there are only a handful of physicians who are presently qualified to enlarge this work, I feel that it is just a matter of time before my basically simple technique becomes widely applied as an important part of the treatment of alcoholism.

5
Physical and Mental Allergies in Children

Are Your Child's Mental and Physical Ailments Allergic Symptoms?

	Yes	No
•Is or was he unable to tolerate his formula?		
•Does or did he break out in rashes or hives?		
•Does or did he have eczema?		
•Does or did he get croup or colic?		
•Is or was vomiting a problem?		
•Does or did he have a stuffy nose, hay fever, asthma, recurrent colds and frequent lower respiratory infections perhaps associated with earaches?		
•Does or did he have facial skin pallor?		
•Does he have dark circles under his eyes?		
•Does he get headaches, stomachaches, growing pains?		
•Does he get "stomach viruses," the "flu," or the "bug" frequently?		
•Does he wet the bed or wet himself during the day?		
•Does he appear depressed or withdrawn?		
•Is he hyperactive or restless?		
•Does he have a short attention span?		

•Do foods (corn, peas, carrots, etc.) appear virtually unchanged in his bowel movements?
•Does he get diarrhea?
•Does he get constipated?
•Is he fatigued or tense?
•Is he learning disabled?
•Is he emotionally unstable?
•Does he crave certain foods?
•Does eating or not eating affect his behavior?
•Does he get carsick?
•Do odors or fumes make him ill?
•Does he love gasoline or paint?

If the answer to any of these questions is "yes," you may well have an allergic child on your hands.

When I was a student at the Long Island College of Medicine I had to make a decision regarding the area in which I would specialize. I had always liked the highly skilled mechanical aspects of surgery, and I appreciated the thinking required in making the types of decisions surgeons must make. In addition I had done very well in my courses in surgery, and so I thought that this would be the area in which I would specialize. But my mind was changed after I encountered the field of pediatrics. The children I saw were so appealing, refreshing, young, and helpless that I felt it was an exciting challenge to make a diagnosis of an infant or a young child (who usually was unable to give any diagnostic information) with a searching, gentle, and skillful examination. After I had obtained the required postgraduate training in pediatrics, I opened an office specializing in the care of infants and children.

During my first years of practice I have to admit that I did not know very much about allergy. My medical school, internship, residency, and early postgraduate courses, along with my clinic work, gave me only a relatively small fund of experience to draw on. Information about problems of this nature was not part of the usual body of information that was acquired during the postgraduate pediatric training. But I did notice I was seeing certain children quite frequently for "chest colds" without fever—noisy "bronchial" infants with rattling chests that I could both hear and feel, and with noses that never seemed to stop running or were always stuffy. In addition, I noticed there was no strong evidence that these children were suffering from infections, since other than being pale, they appeared to be quite well, perhaps a little irritable or restless. I felt that I was dealing with some form of allergy, but I knew very little about this particular specialty or just what was going on in those "bronchial babies" with the stuffy and runny noses. Therefore, my "expertise" in pediatric allergy was limited to simply giving these infants and children safe doses of medication to control their symptoms because I did not know how to eliminate them.

One day in 1953, I read an announcement in the *Journal of the American Medical Association* that Dr. Bret Ratner, one of the original researchers and founding fathers of pediatric allergy, was giving an intensive eight-month course in pediatric allergy at the New York Medical College, and I applied for a place in his course because I hoped that he would be able to provide me with answers to my questions about my young patients.

My association with Dr. Ratner's group was to last for twenty years, and with the passage of time, I became a senior member in the warm fellowship of the pediatric allergy clinic staff, and was appointed assistant professor in the allergy section of the department of pediatrics. At this clinic, for the first time I had an opportunity to observe and work with patients whose ailments were similar to the problems that I had been seeing in my office, but now I was able to do something more than just provide medications for symptoms. We took allergy-oriented histories, studied specimens of nasal and bronchial mucus under the microscope for cellular evidence of allergy, and we performed extensive series of skin tests on every patient. We changed their environments and diets, and we gave desensitizing treatments along with medications. We knew that we must be doing something right because we were able to help many of the children—but not all of them.

There have been many changes in my understanding of allergy which have now led me along paths that are very different from those followed by the fine physicians at New York Medical College with whom I was so pleased to be associated for two decades, but those doctors helped show me the way. And it has been a long and exciting journey of discovery for me from there to the present where I am able to help almost every child I see.

Rule Out Allergies First

It is a rare, most unusual pediatrician who is at all familiar with allergy as a common cause of many problems of infancy and childhood. As a result of this information gap, there are children with unrecognized allergic disorders who have undergone extensive, sometimes very painful, frightening, and often expensive tests that have turned out to be totally unnecessary. Many children have had unnecessary exposure to X-ray radiation of various parts of their bodies with skull X-rays, gastrointestinal (GI) series with fluoroscopy, and barium enemas; electroencephalograms, proctoscopy, cystoscopy; installation of stomach tubes, spinal taps, and anesthesia. There have even been exploratory operations because the condition was of such duration and intensity that surgery appeared to be justified as a proper means of investigation to identify the source of severe and puzzling internal conditions.

About ten years ago while visiting one of my pediatric patients in the hospital I overheard the nurses discussing a seven-year-old child who was going to have a pneumoencephalogram. In this procedure spinal fluid is removed from the lower back and replaced with air so that the chambers and surfaces of the brain are outlined to give what has often proved to be an excellent picture of considerable diagnostic value. In this particular case, the child's physician was concerned that there might possibly be a brain tumor responsible for the headaches, nausea, and vomiting that the child exhibited even though there were no neurological findings present at the time. The pneumoencephalogram is usually followed by a prolonged period of severe headache. I spoke with this youngster for a few minutes and quickly learned that every time he ate eggs he became nauseous, developed cramps, and had severe vomiting! Was it not possible that if eggs could do this to his intestinal tract, that this food-allergic child whose doctor and parents knew he was allergic to eggs might have an undiagnosed allergic headache with associated symptoms of nausea and vomiting on the same basis—food allergy? In my opinion, this child's response to his entire diet and other environmental exposures should have been carefully investigated to determine if other foods or beverages or some types of chemical exposure might be causing him the head pains that were severe enough to justify a pneumoencephalogram. A simple, painless office investigation for bio-ecologic illness and allergy should have been done first. There was no ethical way in which I could make my opinions known. It was necessary for me to remain silent. But a few days later, I learned that the pneumoencephalogram, fortunately, did not show any anatomic abnormalities in the child's brain. Unfortunately, his problem still remained undiagnosed.

If medical students in training and practicing graduate physicians have no understanding of allergy, allergic addiction, chemical susceptibility, and nutritional disturbances, they are not going to understand the nature of such problems when they encounter them. And believe me, they will meet them day after day after day. Allergy will not be suspected or diagnosed in a child with repeated headaches. It is quite possible that, because of the severity of his discomfort, he and his family will be referred to a child guidance center for endless wasted hours of conferences during which various staff members will search in depth and in vain for "social and emotional" factors causing his headaches. They will not have the faintest idea regarding the cause of this child's *reversible, diagnosable,* and *treatable* allergic headache disorder. And while these useless efforts are being made, I have little doubt that many types of drugs will be tried to relieve pain or to tranquilize a nervous system that in fact is an allergic battlefield.

Why a Child Never Really Outgrows His Allergies

For years pediatricians and some traditional allergists have said to the parents of allergic children, "Well, maybe he'll outgrow it." They make this statement because they have observed that as some children grow older, the eggs that used to make them sick no longer seem to cause any problem; the milk they couldn't tolerate no longer seems to affect them adversely, etc.

However, when the now five-year-old child was a carefully controlled, spoon-fed infant, his mother was able to "test" him to see if he could tolerate beef, carrots, rice, bananas, tuna, oats, peas, chicken, etc., one at a time. Now, at age five, he is helping himself to various foods and eating all kinds of food mixtures. If, for instance, he has developed the type of allergy to egg where eating more eggs serves to relieve or cover the allergic withdrawal symptoms caused by a previous meal of egg, his sense of well-being could make egg a favorite food. On the other hand, eating foods containing egg as a hidden food in a mixture, might not produce dramatic symptoms but would keep an allergic state smoldering along. In all these cases, allergy is still present. It is active but just below the surface of awareness—keeping the allergic pot boiling, as it were, causing low-grade chronic symptoms, and permitting the appearance of unexplained flare-ups that the patient, his parents, and physician do not even suspect are related to dietary allergies. There are thousands—hundreds of thousands—of children who have physical and mental problems, who are and will remain ill, uncomfortable, tired, irritable, achy, unproductive, and unhappy, and who never achieve their inherent potential because they are laboring under an allergic burden. Their true nature and their intellectual capacities are clouded over by unsuspected, unrecognized, and incorrectly treated forms of cerebral and "psychosomatic" allergy. These childhood allergies waste many priceless lives that could be salvaged if only practitioners in the healing arts would learn how to diagnose and treat this major threat.

The Feingold Diet for Hyperactive Children

About four years ago, Dr. Benjamin Feingold, a California physician specializing in pediatric allergy, wrote a book for parents of hyperactive (hyperkinetic) and learning-disabled children. Since there are more than 5 million children in the United States who are both learning disabled and hyperactive, I feel it is crucial for me to discuss Dr. Feingold's work in some detail. There are some important areas of fundamental disagreement between us. It has been my experience that the Feingold diet is useful, but it is an *incomplete* approach to the problem of hyperactivity and learning disabilities.

During the past ten years, I have tested many patients for chemical allergy to coal-tar-derived food coloring and artificial flavors by placing various dilutions of yellow, red, or blue FD&C (Food, Drug, and Cosmetic Act) food coloring and a number of artificial flavors under the tongues of my patients. The results have included a wide range of allergic symptoms within a matter of minutes. In his book, Dr. Feingold recommended the elimination of government-certified (coal-tar derived) food coloring and synthetic artificial flavoring agents from children's diets. He, too, noticed that these FD&C food colors and artificial flavors could trigger major personality and behavioral changes in children who were allergic to them. Dr. Feingold's approach to the problem was to have the children follow a special elimination diet for two to three weeks or longer to see if there would be a significant change in behavior and school performance. Sometimes these children improved greatly, other times moderately, and often not at all.

The reason I state that Dr. Feingold's approach is incomplete is because he does not take into account that each food color and artificial flavor is a specific and chemically *unique* material —each having different properties from the other—and some patients may react to some chemicals and not to others. Furthermore, he doesn't take into account that the hyperactive learning disabled children also may be allergic to substances such as the foods they eat and the beverages they drink, including water. Moreover, their highly susceptible nervous systems may react to airborne dusts, pollens, molds, or danders, and other chemical agents that they eat or inhale.

My technicians and I have caused thousands of episodes of symptoms familiar to this group of problem children who are allergic to many substances in addition to food colors and flavors or who are not allergic to any food colors or flavors. It is not unusual to see the following symptoms appear as a result of tests to many different foods, beverages, dust, molds, animal danders, and chemicals: pallor, flushing of the face, hyperactivity, irritability, anger, restlessness, headache, fatigue, abdominal pain, leg muscle pains (typical growing pains), mental confusion, withdrawal, depression, visual blurring, lack of concentration, drowsiness, itching, changes in penmanship, urinary bladder urgency with uncomfortable urination, inability to read, changes in speech, etc. All of these symptoms have been induced in learning-disabled and hyperactive children who, as you can see, have many other problems.

I am in complete agreement with Dr. Feingold's assertion that synthetic food colors and flavorings should be removed from the patient's diet. They are substances foreign to the human body and manufactured in a chemical laboratory—they are not a part of man's natural food supply.

In addition to eliminating food coloring and synthetic flavors, Dr. Feingold suggests foods containing natural salicylates—apricots, prunes, peaches, plums, raspberries, grapes, oranges, cucumbers, tomatoes, and aspirin also be removed from the diet for reasons with which I cannot agree. In his book, *Why Your Child Is Hyperactive,* Dr. Feingold states that allergy to aspirin is a common, serious disorder. On the same page he states that apricots, prunes, peaches, raspberries, grapes, oranges, cucumbers, and tomatoes have the potential to induce the same type of adverse reaction as caused by the manufactured aspirin because they all contain salicylates. Feingold emphasizes the role of salicylate-containing foods, which are an integral part of his program. I have never found a significant correlation between allergy to some of the foods on his list and sensitivity to food colors, flavors, or aspirin. I do not eliminate these foods as a group because each food in and out of the group must be evaluated and incriminated or found negative on an individual basis. This is a broad incrimination with no solid evidence and I cannot accept his speculations versus my direct observations concerning the demonstrable facts in this situation.

However, in the course of one full day of testing at my office, it is often possible to demonstrate the presence or absence of sensitivity to food colors and flavors with a high degree of accuracy. It is not necessary to spend a long period of time waiting to see the effects of the Feingold elimination diet. It is possible to employ simple office procedures and in one day be able to determine whether *any* of the "salicylate" foods or any of the food colorings or flavors were offending agents in the case being investigated.

Asthma and the Parentectomy

Modern medicine has gone too far in the specialty of pediatrics when it permits allergists, pediatricians, and psychiatrists to perform what I consider one of the horrors of the modern era —a parentectomy—where children are exiled to hospitals because their asthma is thought to be the psychosomatic result of parental rejection.

In this form of emotional surgery, asthmatic children and their parents are the unwitting victims of a tragic error on the part of some well-intentioned and seriously misinformed doctors. Because of the many failures that occur in the management of childhood asthma, and because these doctors were not adequately trained in allergy and, therefore, do not know there are *organic* causes for the child's asthma, such as food allergy and chemical susceptibility, well-meaning physicians, impressed by Freudian concepts, conclude that the wheezing in a child's lungs (due to muscular spasm in the bronchial tubes associated with congestion and the accumulation of excessive obstructing mucus) has some *psychiatric* significance. It is claimed that a child somehow becomes aware of maternal rejection and develops asthma as a psychosomatic illness, expressing deep sadness through his lungs because, according to this fairy tale, the brain cannot direct this grief of rejection to the vocal cords. Physicians have come to this inane conclusion even in situations where a mother appears to love her child, states that she loves this child, and in the eyes of all who know her really does seem to love the child.

I am certain that some readers may be shocked by this concept. For some it will be hard to realize that I am not referring to a method of treatment that was employed one hundred years ago and subsequently discarded when it was found to be useless. Parentectomy is a horrible reality—one of the "modern solutions" for the treatment of cases of childhood asthma. We still have among us physicians who believe in and will perform a parentectomy when they are confronted with a difficult case of asthma that cannot be properly managed unless the techniques of bio-ecologic medicine are employed.

These "maternally rejected" children are often sent to special hospitals for "treatment-resistant"* asthmatic children. These hospitals for asthmatic children are located in various parts of the country and are staffed by people of integrity who have dedicated themselves to helping these unfortunate children who suffer from this chronic, at times terribly frightening, and occasionally deadly bio-ecologic disorder of the lower respiratory tract.

When I visited one of these hospitals in the Southeast, the medical director and the administrator were open and friendly and they could not have been nicer. As part of my visit, I inspected the bright and cheerful premises through which they were proud to show me. The hospital was spotlessly clean, but I noted that the floors were freshly waxed, and I could detect the odor of an evaporating petroleum solvent, which was a component of the floor wax.

It disturbed me a great deal to think that such a beautiful, clean, well-equipped, and very well-run institution (established only to help these children) was *chemically polluted*. No one was aware of the fact that the maintenance of this building could be a factor in perpetuating the illness of the patients. The directors and staff probably gave little thought regarding the use of such materials because they did not realize that low concentrations of volatile petrochemical substances are important factors in the genesis of many forms of physical and mental illness, including asthma. Yet, time and time again my col-

---

*The reader should keep in mind that in most cases of asthma the term "treatment-resistant" suggests that the illness really is "untreatable" because it has occurred in a patient who is resisting treatment. This shifts responsibility for failure from the physician to the innocent victim of the illness.

leagues and I have provoked episodes of asthma in children and adults with our tests for allergy (chemical susceptibility) to environmental contamination with the products of modern-day petrochemical technology. The children residing in this beautiful, well-kept facility were repeatedly subjected to a barrage of chemical pollutants that could bring on "unexplained" attacks of asthma. I am sure the ever present environmental chemical stress within this hospital added significantly to the total allergic burden carried by these asthmatic children.

At noon I was invited to the dining room to have lunch with the children and the staff. What would normally be considered a very wholesome meal was provided for the children, but I was disturbed by the fact that all of the children were on the same diet, and food allergy was given only token consideration by not serving eggs, chocolate, fish, nuts, or spices. The dining tables were filled with those foods my colleagues and I have *proved* are major allergic offenders: *Milk, the number-one offender in childhood, was present in large pitchers that were being refilled by a concerned and vigilant staff. Bread, containing wheat, the number-two offender, was freely available to all in generous stacks.* This "wholesome and nutritious" meal consisted of lettuce, tomatoes, potatoes, roast beef, along with bread and milk —all these foods among the most prominent food offenders we have identified as important causes of asthma in asthmatic children.

Why didn't this concerned staff suspect these foods as possible causes for their patients' asthma? Because reactions to foods are often delayed from a few hours to twenty-four hours or longer, and the importance of food allergy, therefore, is not always immediately apparent since the children did not have attacks of asthma during or shortly after eating. No one associated this nutritious food with the appearance of a child's regularly occurring middle-of-the-night or wee-hours-of-the-morning attacks of asthma. Or a child could have a smoldering type of allergic response to a food he is eating frequently and that might be responsible for almost continuous difficulty in breathing throughout the day and night without ever producing recognizable flare-ups that would identify this food as an offender.

In visiting another hospital for asthmatic children in New

York State I was taken on a tour of inspection by the medical administrator and the chief of service. The administrator was a chain smoker,* and I was shocked when he continued to smoke after leaving his office. As we went from room to room and ward to ward, he continued to light up and smoke one cigarette after another. This man, who kept all the machinery of the hospital running smoothly, was continuously polluting the air with tobacco smoke from which the children could not escape. The chief of service, a board-certified allergist, also seemed oblivious to the great clouds of smoke produced by his administrator. In addition to the tobacco smoke, there was another serious chemical problem. During the inspection tour I noted the very strong odor of a deodorizing disinfectant that was applied liberally in each of the bathrooms. The chemical fumes from this disinfectant burned my eyes slightly and caused a minor irritation in my throat. I have seen many patients who were made violently ill by disinfectant fumes, and I have no doubt that this additional chemical pollution in the bathrooms that was also drifting in the air of the hospital corridors and rooms throughout the building was hurting these children terribly.

I did not discuss my concerns with the staff members of the hospital because I had not come to their institution as a consultant. I was a guest, and my hosts practiced *conventional* medicine. I know that they believed they were doing the right things to help these children. They certainly were very kind to their patients; there was an atmosphere of genuine affection and warmth in these institutions. I was impressed by the fact that my colleagues were decent human beings who were doing their best. I remained silent with the unspoken thought that they had a lot to learn about the causes of the illness they were treating.

Of course, there are some children who do improve shortly after leaving their parents and entering a hospital—not because the doctors performed a "parentectomy," but because they performed an "environmentectomy." The child is separated not only from his parents, but from some of the foods, bever-

---

*Bronchial allergy to tobacco smoke is so common that at least 20 to 50 percent of the asthmatic children who were patients in this hospital could not possibly have gotten better.

ages, molds, pollens, dusts, danders, and chemicals that were in his home environment! Environmental stresses were eliminated! The chemically susceptible child's health greatly improves because he is no longer sleeping in a bedroom located above the garage from which gas and oil fumes seeped into his bedroom and were an important factor in his asthmatic condition. In addition, he is separated from the home that is chemically polluted by his mother's housekeeping procedures, which employ chlorinated cleansers and bleaches, furniture and floor polishes, room deodorizers, and insect sprays; by his father's after-shave lotion and cigarette smoking; by his sister's hobby materials, which include glues, paints, lacquers, and varnishes; and he is no longer exposed to the combustion fumes generated when natural gas is burned in the kitchen stove, oven, clothes dryer, water heater and hot-air heating system of his home.

Is it any wonder that there are times when my colleagues and I feel that we are voices crying in the wilderness? Those of us who practice bio-ecologic medicine and understand the true nature and scope of allergy have had many successes in the management of "treatment-resistant" cases of asthma in children and adults. I have seen dozens of asthmatic patients in my office who were told elsewhere that their allergic bronchial disorders were due to emotional causes. So far I have been able to prove the diagnoses 100 percent wrong. Of course, there may be a few children whose family relationships constitute an unbearable burden of psychic stress; life in their particular households may very well be an emotional nightmare with which they are unequipped to cope but, in every case of so-called "intrinsic" asthma, I have found the polluted home or unrecognized food allergy are the important factors.

A severe case of asthma requires very careful hospital supervision, and at times it is necessary to have the services of a well-trained pulmonary physiologist available in case there are any violent flare-ups of the asthmatic symptoms as the patient travels the road to recovery. At the present time, I know of only three hospitals where a program of comprehensive environmental control can be followed. They are the American International Hospital in Zion, Illinois, where Dr. Randolph is located; the Brooklawn Hospital in Dallas, Texas, where Dr.

William Rea practices; and St. Mary's Hospital in Port Arthur, Texas, where Dr. Harris Hosen employs this technique. I have sent some of my most difficult cases to these three highly qualified colleagues and friends, and each of them performed a remarkable human-salvage operation in the worst cases I have seen.

CASE STUDY: HYPERACTIVITY/HEADACHES/SHORT-TERM MEMORY LOSS/ALLERGIC PSEUDO-RETARDATION

Allergic symptoms can take many forms in children. I coined the term "allergic pseudo-retardation" because I have seen some children with bio-ecologic mental illness who are very intelligent and yet function at levels far below their capacity. In addition to these talented underachievers, there are children of average ability who appear to be considerably below average or retarded. I define allergic pseudo-retardation as a mental condition occurring in a child who is not "permanently" retarded because of genetic factors or a previous brain injury but gives the impression that he is retarded because of cerebral malfunction which makes it impossible for his allergic brain to perform normally. The definition of my term, nutritional or allergic pseudo-retardation, is self-evident.

A nine-year old boy, Chris H., was brought to me because his aunt, a teacher who specializes in the education of children with learning disabilities, had attended a symposium at the New York Institute for Child Development where she recognized the problems of many of her students in the presentation that I was invited to give. Chris was described as being an anxious and tense little boy. He had great difficulty with his penmanship and formed letters poorly. A learning disabilities specialist who studied his problem concluded that he was suffering from a "short-term memory defect," which made him unable to remember or reproduce the shape of written letters of the alphabet as well as he should have at age nine.

As I listened to Chris solve a problem, it was obvious that he was a very intelligent child. His method of reaching an answer was impressive to anyone observing this process because of the large amount of collateral knowledge he had to retrieve from his memory and assess to formulate his answer. Bright as he was, he was mentally handicapped because he could not give a prompt answer to a simple question that required information that should have been instantly available to him "at his finger-tips."

During our initial consultation, in which I carefully reviewed certain aspects of his past history, a number of significant facts were obtained that suggested a number of factors that might have caused his penmanship difficulties and underachievement at school. The following information has been selected from my office records to illustrate the type of data that can be obtained if one asks the right questions regarding the effects of food, beverages, chemicals, and substances naturally present in the atmosphere:

Chocolate: Chris had had abdominal pains of moderate severity followed by several loose bowel movements almost every time plain chocolate was eaten during the past eight years. Small amounts of chocolate appeared to be well tolerated and he often ate brownies, chocolate ice cream, chocolate pudding, and a chocolate-flavored breakfast cereal.

Apple cider vinegar: Each time Chris was exposed to the odor of vinegar he immediately got a headache in his lower forehead; he is very fond of apples from which cider vinegar is prepared.

Lateness for a meal: He would get a headache, which is one of the characteristic withdrawal symptoms of food addiction. Usually this late-for-meal headache was greatly relieved by his favorite cherry-flavored red gelatin dessert, which contains artificial coloring, synthetic flavoring and sugar. His withdrawal headaches could be partially relieved by a chocolate-flavored cold cereal with milk. These were the only specific factors in his diet that were capable of relieving a headache that resulted from not eating on time.

Petrochemicals and coal-tar derivatives: Chris would have symptoms within a few minutes after exposure to a number of volatile substances. Fumes from plastic cement used in model making, airplane glue, and the exhaust from diesel engines caused a severe headache; hair spray caused itching and burning of his eyes; tobacco smoke would bring about moderately severe coughing. He also mentioned that detergents have a "bad" smell and rubber has a "good" smell. Observations of this type are often made by patients who are susceptible to environmental chemicals.

Using the information I obtained from the history of his reactions to foods and environmental chemicals, I began a series of sublingual tests (placing small quantities of different test solutions under his tongue) to observe the bodywide effects of various foods and chemicals. Here are some of the reactions that were obtained from these tests:

Chocolate: Mental confusion, impaired memory, and deterioration of penmanship and spelling, which was then followed by increased mental alertness and an amazing change in his penmanship when the dose of the chocolate-testing solution was changed and his symptoms (due to chocolate reactions, from which he never was free) were neutralized. His usual penmanship was characterized by large letters that were fairly well formed; the words were spread out horizontally with errors in spelling. It was evaluated as being at the performance level of a seven-year-old second-grade student. The neutralizing dose of chocolate extract made him alert and cleared the "allergic" dysfunctions in his brain and neuromuscular system that were causing his poor penmanship (dysgraphia). A neutralizing dose of chocolate extract changed his penmanship from that of a second-grade student to that of a third-or fourth-grade student within a matter of minutes.

Apple: He became restless and irritable, with facial flushing, and moderately tired. During this reaction he made a number of errors in spelling and his fatigue increased; he had to rest his head on the desk.

Milk: Chris became hyperactive, made errors in spelling, and his usually poor handwriting became worse. He then exhibited paranoid behavior and hyperactivity which required physical restraint because it appeared that he might injure others in the testing laboratory.

Petrochemical ethyl alcohol: He became extremely tired with flushing of his face and ears. Next he complained of abdominal pains and became restless, swinging his legs back and forth, and said that he just had to get outside. He had to leave the office.

Red food coloring (FD&C Red #2): This coal-tar product made Chris irritable and restless; his face and ears became flushed. He was unable to concentrate on reading, began to argue, and once again became aggressive, hostile, and paranoid and expressed a desire to leave the office and go outside.

Symptoms That Come and Go

It is usually possible to determine the probable causes of many disorders that are characterized by a fairly constant and predictable pattern of symptoms or follow a particular time schedule or occur in a specific geographic location. In most instances, something useful can be learned about an illness that fluctuates in intensity and in which the symptoms may vary from mild to severe or perhaps disappear completely, then return unpredictably—out of the blue. The fact that the disease can disappear, leaving its victim symptom-free for a matter of minutes, hours, or days, is impressive evidence that the condition is reversible and there is no *permanent damage* at the sites where the illness localizes or it would not be possible for the symptoms to clear up completely. Problems do not disappear mysteriously even though it seems as if they do so; the responsible factors have not been identified and patients are unaware of which exposures might be causing their condition. Normal functions are being interfered with by controllable identifiable external factors.

A child whose penmanship is very poor may occasionally have much better handwriting, which is wrongly attributed to a "real effort" or "a desire to please," and poor penmanship is often unjustly misinterpreted as being a manifestation of carelessness, laziness, or lack of interest or of a desire to do well. A similar situation exists with respect to children whose reading ability is generally poor to fair yet who, on occasion, may do remarkably better for brief periods of time. The "experts" do not realize that *any* good performance *proves* that there is an ability or capacity to do well which is being seriously interfered with by a reversible brain dysfunction that may be present most of the time. "Reading disability," "dyslexia," "perceptual disorder," and "minimal brain dysfunction" are descriptive diagnoses that conceal the experts' lack of knowledge regarding the underlying cause of the problems confronting them.

Many adults forget that a child's primary occupation is the serious business of being a student, and there are very few children who really do not want to perform well at school. Allergically reacting youngsters who suffer from chronic or frequent episodes of cerebral and body dysfunctions simply cannot be good students. No matter how great their desire to succeed, they are doomed to failure if they operate in a milk or wheat fog of confusion, depression, restlessness, or irritability—a fog that never lifts so long as they eat without knowledge of the cerebral effects of common offenders to which they are exposed several times a day. If it's not the diet, cerebral and body functions may be impaired by a chemical cloud that always surrounds them at home or in school.

I cannot accept the concept that a "damaged brain" will malfunction sometimes and perform normally at other times, unless those who employ the term "damaged" mean that a normal brain is temporarily malfunctioning. This normal brain, which is part of the body of a susceptible individual, will perform as if it were damaged when it reacts after an exposure to some offending environmental agent(s) to which it is susceptible. Many specialists who employ the terms "minimal brain damage" (MBD) and "minimal brain dysfunction" (MBD) really do not think about the basic implications of these terms. It is obvious that if academic performance and behavior are not normal, we have some malfunction of the brain and nervous system but the symptoms are merely noted as a dysfunction of the brain. They are catalogued but not understood. If a brain is intermittently malfunctioning, obviously something is temporarily wrong with it at times, and to designate this condition as MBD is correct. Unfortunately, this is where most specialists in the area of learning disabilities, with its often associated hyperactivity, end or limit their thinking on this subject. Much more is demanded of the "experts" here. They cannot lightly pass over or ignore the nature of this reversible damage which does not constitute permanent injury of the brain tissue. Damage is presumed to be due to some minimal injury that occurred during birth. I know experimental studies with young animals that were deprived of oxygen have shown that they have poor mental performance as compared with their litter mates. I know that a small number of such birth-injured children do exist. But because there are such children, along with some unfortunate youngsters who have deformities of their nervous system, we cannot overlook the fact that most of the children who are so diagnosed are suffering from reversible allergic and nutritional disorders whose causes can be identified and eliminated or controlled.

CASE STUDY: EPILEPSY

One of the interesting observations made by the father of one of my patients having seizures was the fact that her convulsions always occurred on Mondays and had done so for six or seven consecutive weeks. In reviewing the patient's daily activities and diet, the outstanding factor to emerge was that it had recently become the family habit to go to a nut and candy store known as the Nut House every Sunday. To me it seemed more than coincidence that the Monday seizures began about the time that this patient started eating a rather large quantity of peanuts on each of these Sunday visits.

A simple ecologic procedure was followed, namely, the patient was removed from her dietary environment. The weekly trips to the Nut House were discontinued on Sunday and her Monday convulsions promptly disappeared. Several other interesting observations were made in this case. Both parents had noted that this eight-year-old girl often would have a flushed face in the early evening of those nights during which she would have a seizure, which was characterized by jerking movements of her arms. There were other nights when she had similar seizures that did not follow the appearance of redness in her face.

A sublingual (under the tongue) test with tomato extract produced facial flushing in the office, and there were several other foods that caused symptoms but no seizures were reproduced during testing. The patient was placed on a seven-day Rotary Diversified Diet and her parents were instructed to make detailed notes concerning any observations that they felt might be significant. On our next consultation within a month, the patient's father presented me with a chart of daily information which in many ways was like a mathematical solution to a puzzle. The ingestion of tomato was followed by facial flushing, and later on each of the evenings when tomato was eaten, the patient had her typical seizures. It was also clearly evident that apples or apple juice also produced seizure activity.

CASE STUDY: GEORGE BALLENTINE*—NAUSEA/ABDOMINAL PAIN/HEADACHE/DIZZINESS/SCHOOL PROBLEMS

George Ballentine is a pleasant and very likable fifteen-year-old boy who came to my office with his parents in March 1977. Although he was bright, well adjusted, and socially active in school, he was unable to attend classes because he had severe abdominal pains, nausea, headache, and spells of dizziness. He had been absent from school, especially during the months of January, February and March, during the past three years due to his illness.

In reviewing his past history, his mother told me that George had had colic for the first three months of his life. At age nine he was admitted to the local hospital in Pennsylvania because he was "run down" and suffering from headaches, dizziness, and what was described as the "flu." He was discharged from the hospital without any diagnosis. At age eleven, the abdominal pains started and the next year the chronic headaches began. By the time he was fifteen, the abdominal pains had localized in the lower mid-abdomen above the pubic area, and 50 percent of the time they were associated with an urge to have a bowel movement. Since age eleven he had had these symptoms almost every day, and sometimes at night the pain would wake him and cause him to double up in agony. Each episode would last from five to ten minutes. The pains would build up to a peak, decrease in intensity, and return again. Abdominal

*This informative case history is reported with the kind permission of George's parents as a public service to help others with similar problems.

pain usually appeared about one hour after eating—especially after breakfast or after his bedtime snack. During the month prior to his visit with me, he had been getting headaches twice a day which localized in the back of his head and were characterized by pressure and throbbing.

His "chemical" history was typical for an individual suffering from chemical allergies. Polystyrene glue used for bonding plastics in model making made him dizzy, he couldn't stand the odor of permanent felt-tipped markers, and he would have severe nausea after an exposure to hair spray or the odor of a new car. In a room where people were smoking cigarettes, his nose would run and his eyes would burn and tear—his level of discomfort was such that he had to leave the room. He liked the odor of gasoline and loved that of freshly printed newspapers and the fumes from duplicator fluid employed in the ditto process. He hated the odor of fresh tar and newly applied asphalt; he did not become ill from this exposure but noted that "somehow" they bothered him. There was a high level of air pollution in his immediate environment. There were four oil wells located three hundred feet (the minimum legal distance) from the property line of his home, and natural gas was being burned on the top of three of them. In foggy weather, everyone in the neighborhood could smell "gas" and crude oil; gas fumes frequently escaped from these wells and often were not burned off at the top.

While George was visiting my office in Connecticut, just being away from his home town decreased his symptoms considerably. When I brought this observation to his parents' attention, they mentioned that when George went to visit his aunt in another town, his symptoms cleared up after being in her home for three days. It was apparent that his home and school environment were important factors in the health of this extremely chemically susceptible young man who was experiencing massive exposures.

After obtaining the details of his highly informative history, George's testing program began. It is important to remember that he arrived at the Alan Mandell Center with a headache that had been present for twenty-four hours.

Ethanol (synthetic petroleum-derived alcohol): The first test decreased his headache slightly. The second dose gave an urge to sneeze and the third dose increased his headache; he also passed gas from his lower bowel and began to belch. The fourth test dose completely eliminated his headache. *Comment:* Because I strongly suspected that petroleum products were a major cause of his symptoms, I asked my chief technician to give George various doses of ethanol to see if she could determine a neutralizing dose that would decrease or eliminate his headache.

Rice: He developed severe, dull generalized headache, which began in the back of his head, and very sharp abdominal pains. *Comment:* Rice is mistakenly considered by many allergists to be "the" hypoallergenic food, and they often recommend it as a diet staple to many allergic individuals. About 60 percent of the patients I have tested for sensitivity to rice have reacted to it, and in this case rice was one of George's most frequently eaten foods.

Lamb: He passed a great deal of gas through his lower bowel and had severe abdominal cramps, as well as sharp pain in the back of his head.

Milk: Dizziness developed, eyes teared.

Tuna: This, too, made him dizzy. He had a headache over his right eye and in the back of his head, with moderately severe throbbing in the left temple.

Honey: Patient sneezed, had extreme fatigue and put his head on the desk. Headache developed in back of head.

Pineapple: Sharp pain occurred over his right eye. He had moderately severe abdominal pain and was passing gas from his lower bowel, associated with a sudden painful urge to have a bowel movement. He said that he felt "like a bomb was going to explode in his abdomen."

Yellow food coloring: Abdominal "gas" pains developed.

Tomato: No reaction.

Corn: No reaction.

House dust from Center Laboratory: No reaction.

House dust from Endo Laboratory: Patient had headache, dizziness.

Broccoli: George sneezed, had a runny nose, was slightly dizzy.

Mixed grass pollens: No reaction.

Mixed weed pollens: Patient became moderately irritable, edgy, slightly dizzy. He had a dull ache in upper forehead.

Mixed tree pollens: This produced very severe pressure in back of head, moderate facial flushing, dizziness, inability to concentrate.

Squash: He became very confused, unable to concentrate, slightly dizzy. *Comment:* Squash, like rice, is another one of those presumed benign (hypoallergenic) foods that are just as capable of causing important reactions in a sensitive patient as any of the other food offenders that are widely recognized.

Cantaloupe: He became very confused, unable to concentrate, fatigued. *Comment:* Cantaloupe is a close botanic relative to squash; they are members of the gourd family. It is interesting to note that in this patient each food affected his nervous system in almost the same way. The fact that the foods are closely related is suggestive, but one cannot conclude without testing, that he would have reacted to both foods. He might not have had any response to cantaloupe, or he could have had entirely different symptoms, such as joint pains, abdominal cramps, or itching. In addition, canteloupe usually has a considerable quantity of mold growing on it that could cause reactions.

Vegetable garden spray: Nausea and belching followed.

Auto exhaust: Pressure developed in back of head, as well as dizziness, sniffles.

Black pepper: Moderately severe dull aching in left abdomen.

Toothpaste: Sneezing and belching followed.

Vinegar: Patient had sharp stomach cramps, sudden urge to move his bowels. (He ran to the bathroom.) Moderately severe occipital pressure headache and restlessness developed. We had to give him oxygen to relieve him.

Alternaria (mold): Occipital (back of the head) headache.

Aspergillus (mold): Headache. Slight dizziness.

Hormodendrum (mold): No reaction.

Penicillium (mold): Pressure in the back of his head.

Stemphyllium (mold): Slight occipital headache.

Tricophyton (mold): Pressure over the eyes, lower forehead, and back of head. Slightly dizzy. Eyes hurt when he moved them and looked from side to side.

George immediately began a Rotary Diversified Diet from which all test-identified offending foods were eliminated. I started a series of desensitizing treatments for dust, molds, respiratory tract bacteria, tree pollens, grass pollens, and weed pollens. At home his parents initiated an environmental control program that included disconnecting the gas stove, removing various chemical agents from the basement, keeping the car out of the garage, which was right under his bedroom, and scrubbing the oil drippings from the garage floor so that the fumes from this material could not penetrate his bedroom above. They also discovered and repaired a defect in the combustion chamber of the gas heating system in their home.

George came to my office on March 11, 1977; testing was started immediately and we began his treatment and environmental control on March 14, after four days of consultation and testing. On March 25, I received a note from his mother stating "George has been free of abdominal cramping except for one single two-hour period after he got his first desensitizing treatment." (Treatment material contains allergenic extracts of the substances the person is sensitive to. It is not unusual for patients to experience some of their familiar symptoms during the early phase of treatment as each individual program is developed and the illness begins to come under control.)

In August, his mother sent me the following note:

Unbeknownst to George, gasoline spilled on the garage floor under his bedroom late at night. Wiped it up. Floor not scrubbed. George awoke in the morning with severe headache, abdominal pain, and gas. After being out of the house for two hours, he cleared up. We have made the following observations:

Tar: George helped with roof on the house. Had to quit because of headache and dizziness.

Turpentine: Used for five minutes, nauseous and lethargic for several hours even though he left the room immediately.

Paste wax for furniture: Not thinking, I used this with George present. Within minutes he had severe abdominal pain and was passing gas. He left the area and was fine in thirty minutes.

Exhaust fumes: We had him try mowing the lawn (gasoline mower) at the beginning of the summer, and the same symptoms that occurred with furniture wax occurred within fifteen minutes. The

odor of freshly mowed grass which released grass terpenes caused
him to have confusion, headache, dizziness, and nausea.

Weather: When it is extremely humid, he still has the same problem
—apparently the gas from the surrounding oil wells is being held
close to the ground.

Gas fumes: The Youth Fellowship had a week-long fair again this year.
George and I were helping by making sandwiches at the fair. We'd
been working only a short time when, for no apparent reason,
George angrily threw a handful of lettuce on the floor, saying, "I'm
not making any more dumb subs!" I was working across the table
from him and I asked him to empty our three cans of water. He
said, "What water?" I told him to bring the green pail he was
standing beside. This time I noticed that his eyes showed confusion and disorientation. I said, "George, you are so confused you
don't even know where you are, do you?" He said he knew where
he was, but I had to tell him again to empty the water in the rest
room. About an hour later, it dawned on me what had caused this
strange behavior: They had begun to operate a gas-fired kiln in
one of the displays, and the fans drew the gas fumes into our
building! I felt terrible because I had been so short with him. After
he "cleared" he was back working as hard as ever. The next morning I apologized for saying what I had said to him. *And he didn't
remember the incident.* [Author's emphasis.] He didn't remember
throwing the lettuce and walking away from the assembly line. As
a rule, he is quite willing to do his share. And is conscientious about
doing it right. [Author's comment: This is a typical instance of
"allergic amnesia."]

He told me he is afraid this will happen in school again this year.
I tried to reassure him now that we know the causes, all or much
of it can be prevented.

I was concerned about the chemical exposures to be encountered when George returned to school. The environmental
problems under consideration were air-polluting oil wells
located close to his home and the chemical agents used in school
for maintenance. I could have recommended homebound in-
struction, but I felt that this would probably not be enough even
though he usually felt more comfortable at home. In addition,
he should have the social contacts that school offered. In an

attempt to resolve this problem, I wrote the following note to his school:

To Whom It May Concern:

George is a patient of mine and his case is extremely complex. He is very sensitive to petrochemicals and coal-tar derivatives such as: gasoline, tar, waxes, polishes, turpentine, solvents, detergents, plastics, oil, paints, disinfectants, rubber, sprays, and alcohol. They cause nausea, cramping, lethargy, and an inability to concentrate. I have been informed that George has experienced problems at school because of his sensitivities and reactions following exposures. His mother has investigated his situation and has determined that many of the cleaning agents used in school contained such substances as alcohol, solvents, penetrants, detergents, polyethylene, deodorizers, etc. to which George reacts.

I was very pleased to learn that your school has been cooperating in every way to help George. I hope that this much appreciated cooperation will be continued to the utmost so that with your kind and absolutely necessary assistance, this young man can comfortably settle down to his studies.

On September 9, 1977, another letter from George's mother:

I am writing regarding George. . . . School opened yesterday and he had problems after being there less than three hours. Once again the pressure in the back of his head returned and turned into a severe headache and pressure behind the eyes. As the day progressed, he became confused and extremely tired. It was an effort to walk up the stairs to the second floor by the end of the day. The school officials were aware of his problem and prepared his schedule to keep him away from all shop, science, and art areas. [Author's note: In my experience this is an unusual degree of understanding, concern, and cooperation on the part of a school.] I contacted the school psychologist and told him what had taken place because he has worked with us for the past years. He said it points more than ever to the agents used by the custodial staff because there were no science labs or such yesterday.
. . .

We are working with the vice-principal and the guidance counselor. They have asked George to keep a diary each day at fifteen-minute intervals to pinpoint his location when the symptoms appear. If they set a pattern, they will change his routes through the hallways, and the classrooms he is assigned to if necessary. School officials are really trying. . . .

Unfortunately for George, his school experience did not improve sufficiently despite the effort of those wonderful school personnel. I received another letter from his mother stating that one night George asked her if he could have a talk with her. She wrote:

George started to talk and cry. He said he couldn't go back to school because he said, "I won't be back more than three weeks and I'll feel terrible again. It has happened in the past three years. I feel fine. Then it gets to the point where I can't stand the confusion, the crowding, the noise, the competition. I feel like I have been ready to flip out for the past three years. And I have been afraid to tell you about it." On further questioning, he said he had looked forward to going back to school with high hopes that that year would be different. Now he had to force himself to go to school. I told him he had done a good job of covering up. And he said, "That's just what it has been—a coverup."

The next letter from Mrs. Ballentine indicated that despite George's improvement because of desensitization, dietary control, and environmental precautions, they had finally made the decision to uproot and move away from the oil wells. Mrs. Ballentine asked my opinion regarding an income tax deduction based on the necessity of a "forced" move for health reasons. I told her she must discuss it with her accountant or lawyer. According to Mrs. Ballentine, the local IRS office initially said no, but at the same time, they were quite vague about it. My letter to Mrs. Ballentine went as follows:

There is no doubt that your home environment is partially responsible for George's health problems, and it is recommended that you provide him with an environment that is as free as possible from chemical agents, molds, etc. George obviously reacts to factors in your home environment in an adverse fashion after only a short exposure. A controlled environment is essential for his health.

It is possible that we can increase his tolerance for some of the things to which he is now allergic by the time he reaches adulthood. There is probably very little chance that this will happen if his present environment continues to aggravate his condition, undermines his general state of health, and prevents him from mobilizing the necessary defenses he must have in operation if he is to recover and lead a normal life.

Mrs. Ballantine also asked me if I knew of any school anywhere in the United States that was designed and operated for children with bio-ecologic illness. Unfortunately, I had to say no. Hopefully, the no-smoking religious college in rural Pennsylvania, which was well tolerated by one of my schizophrenic patients, Jennifer, will still be available in the future if we can just get this very nice young man successfully through high school. In the interim, the Ballentines moved a short distance away from the oil fields, and George experienced the same improvement he felt when staying at his aunt's house.

CASE STUDY: LAURA BELANGER*—"BRAIN DAMAGE"/LEARNING DISABILITIES/HYPERACTIVITY AND HYPOACTIVITY

Laura Belanger had been diagnosed as being hypoactive (sluggish) and hyperactive. When Laura was brought to me, her mother said that Laura was physically sluggish, it was "unnatural" for her to hurry, and her balance was poor. Also, Laura often would lose her train of thought while she was talking, had difficulty dressing herself, and when she was doing something, often forgot what it was she was doing. According to her mother, Laura seemed to move in "slow motion" all the time. She was poorly oriented—often went the wrong direction to return to her classroom and got lost in school. Three to four nights each week Laura was kept awake by severe itching, and her skin showed many typical linear scabs which were caused by her frequent scratching, but there was no visible rash from any skin condition that could have made her itch. Although Laura had a series of negative urine tests, there were problems with bladder control, and she had a need to urinate frequently.

*This interesting and important case history is reported with the kind permission of Laura's family, who believe they may be able to help other children by sharing their experiences with other parents. On behalf of those who will benefit from this information, I thank these good people for making the road to recovery an easier path for others to follow because of their kindness.

A letter, dated January 1977, from Laura's teacher contained the following comments:

Her coordination is average in the use of pencils and crayons. She has some difficulty using scissors. She seems to do her best work early in the morning. After lunch she is tired and listless. She seems content to sit and watch others or daydream. Her response to an oral command is slow to sluggish to reluctant. If you ask her to take out her books, she may respond with a blank look on her face. If she is coloring, she continues to color, and appears not to have heard you talking to her, and I have to get the book for her. Usually she is by herself. When asked why she doesn't play with the other children she says they are mean to her.

Because of her unresponsiveness, she is receiving the brunt of a lot of remarks which affect her enough to make her cry. Children call her a "retard" because of the blank look on her face and her inability to engage in the task at hand.

I found her to be of average ability but she needs a one-to-one learning situation before she responds. [Author's note: In 1975, on her Stanford Binet test, Laura's IQ was 120—which is superior.] She is in a reading group with one other girl. She was placed in a larger reading group, but I found her pinching the child next to her, kicking his shoes, playing with her reading book by putting it on her head, or staring off into space.

According to Laura's school psychologist, on "good" days, Laura was energetic and didn't require much time to complete tasks, and performed with greater ease and efficiency. On "bad" days, she'd dawdle, get tired easily, and was not as able to focus her attention. She spoke constantly in the manner of a younger child. Her vocabulary, however, was superior. Her language was unusual though. She would say things like "I can't get my feet watch. Towels are really blankets. Patches—I mean, purses . . . I can't get the word." Like many children suffering from bio-ecologic illness, Laura's history was characterized by variability of symptoms. Her writing was sometimes neat and normal in appearance with the letters well shaped. On other occasions, Laura's penmanship was written in reverse (if you held it up to a mirror you could read it). She had a large vocabulary, but she could not seem to put the words together. All these are symptoms suggestive of a serious disorder of her nervous system.

In continuing our initial discussion, Laura's mother told me that when the weather became damp, Laura's schoolwork suffered terribly. This suggested two possibilities to me. It could be related to the tremendous increase in the number of atmospheric molds during damp weather (molds thrive and reproduce rapidly in dampness), or it could be related to air pollution. Pollutants are trapped by the humidity and kept close to the ground, giving an increased exposure to pollutants and molds. As I pursued the subject, Mrs. Belanger told me Laura had had an allergic reaction in the past to penicillin. She had been unable to sleep and had had a flare-up of her urinary symptoms, passing urine frequently and without control, which caused her to wet herself. Her nervous system had also become involved in the penicillin reaction, and she had become so unsteady that she had to hold her mother's hand for support.

When I reviewed Laura's history in detail regarding foods, beverages, inhalants, and chemicals, I learned that Laura had a craving for sweets that was so intense that when she was on a restricted diet, she actually cried for them. On shopping trips, Laura fought with her mother and would scream in supermarkets until she was given some candy. Milk caused Laura abdominal pain. On the one or two occasions Laura was permitted a sip of wine or beer, she fell down. Laura gets nauseous, develops abdominal pain, and wants the window open when riding in the family car.

The results of her testing were fascinating. Here are some of them:

Milk: Milk is the number-one offender in children—the cause of many mental, physical, and "psychosomatic" ailments. When Laura was tested with a few drops of milk extract (which were placed under her tongue) she had a series of hiccups and then her penmanship changed. She reversed the letters L and B in her first and last names as shown on page 164.

Wheat: Although wheat is the number-two offender in children, Laura showed no reaction to this cereal grain. This was an important negative test which acted as a control.

Sugar: Her face became slightly flushed and she developed generalized itching with hiccups. (Remember, Laura was waking up at
night with severe itching and this was a very serious complaint for
which no one could find a cause.)

Eggs: She developed a sore throat and generalized itching.

Orange: Orange is a major allergic offender in many people, but Laura
did not have any reaction to it. This test also served as a control.

Apple: This produced moderately severe itching.

Vinegar: This produced vaginal itching. Now we have three causes
(sugar, eggs, and apple) for her itching, and this information was
gathered in the early phase of testing. The vinegar employed in
this test was apple cider vinegar.

Potato: She had a slight stomachache from the first dose, and after the
second dose she had an impairment of memory and could not
remember her middle name. She also developed a moderately
severe sore throat. Laura ate potato frequently, and this test
demonstrated that her respiratory tract, gastrointestinal tract, and
brain were involved in reactions to this food.

   Comment: If people who are allergic to potatoes eat them two
or three times a week, they will never be free of reaction to this
food. Perhaps on the day that Laura ate potatoes or on the day
after, she would have difficulty in school. As the effect started to
wear off and she began to perform a little better, she would eat
potatoes again; and no one would every know why there was an
irregularity in her school performance. To me, irregularity in performance—and I feel that I cannot emphasize this fact enough—
is almost a guarantee that the problem at hand is reversible. Although at times it takes a great deal of effort and patience, in most
instances we should be able to identify the causes of a schoolchild's
irregular behavior.

Peanut: Laura loved peanut butter, and when tested with peanut
extract she became extremely restless and silly; she kept laughing
inanely. She exhibited what her mother called "typical" hyperactivity.

Auto exhaust: Laura promptly got a stomachache, which dovetailed
with her history of having abdominal pain and nausea while riding
in the family car. She did not know she was being tested with
automobile exhaust, but her car-related symptoms were reproduced.

PENMANSHIP CHANGES (DETERIORATION) AND SYMPTOMS INDUCED BY SUBLINGUAL TESTING FOODS AND MOLDS

LAURA BELANGER   **AGE 7**

PRESENTING COMPLAINTS: LEARNING DISABILITIES, LOSS OF EQUILIBRIUM, ENURESIS, INTERMITTENT HYPERACTIVITY AND HYPOACTIVITY

PATIENT'S USUAL PENMANSHIP   *Laura Belanger*

POTATO   PATIENT WAS UNABLE TO REMEMBER HER MIDDLE NAME. SHE EXPERIENCED PHARYNGEAL PAIN AND ABDOMINAL PAIN.

Laura Belanger

MILK   PATIENT HICCUPED FREQUENTLY.

Jaura Belnger

REVERSAL OF "L" AND "B," OMISSION OF "n"

Jaura Elglanger

REVERSAL OF "L," "B," AND "e"

PEANUT   PATIENT BECAME SILLY WITH UNCONTROLLED LAUGHTER.

Laura 'Belanger

FUSARIUM   PATIENT EXPERIENCED EXTREME HYPERACTIVITY. "THIS
mold   IS WHY WE ARE HERE" WAS THE MOTHER'S COMMENT.

Laura Belonger

REVERSAL OF "a" IN LAST NAME

Belang er

REVERSAL OF "e"

ASPERGILLUS   PATIENT BECAME CRANKY, UNCOOPERATIVE, AND FRUSTRATED
mold   HER TONGUE AND NECK BECAME EXTREMELY ITCHY.

Lauranger

PATIENT COMBINED HER FIRST AND SECOND NAMES

Ethanol (synthetic ethyl alcohol prepared from petroleum): Laura developed a stomachache.

Malt: She was tested for malt because a few sips of beer made her fall down, and she was eating malt-containing breakfast cereal. Her tongue burned and her throat became moderately sore.

Comment: This explains why many individuals who seek medical attention for a sore throat may be told after examination that their throat looks normal and the doctor is quite puzzled by the intensity of the patient's discomfort. I had a personal experience with this phenomenon many years ago with a sore throat that bothered me for six weeks. I saw an excellent ear, nose, and throat specialist, who examined me on a number of occasions during that six-week period and found nothing wrong, although I was having moderately severe discomfort every day. This was my first experience with pain in a normal-appearing throat.

In contrast, during testing for allergy, I have produced instant sore throats that are bright red in appearance within just a few minutes after the patient has been tested. Such a throat would have been misdiagnosed as a streptococcus infection by many physicians because of the pain and typical bright red appearance of the tissues. Frequent sore throats are not necessarily due to infections, but in order to protect the patient's best interests, one must always rule out the possibility of infection before diagnosing probable allergy. I know that thousands of tonsils have been sacrificed because of allergic sore throats that can imitate strep infections. Tonsils have often been removed from children and adults having a "tendency" to get sore throats. The tendency to having throat involvement was there but the sore throats were not chronic or recurrent respiratory infections in these allergic individuals.

Chlorine: (This test was done because she was drinking chlorinated tap water at home.) Her tongue burned, she got a moderately sore throat, and felt as if something were burning the lining of her nose. Then she became hyperactive and very silly. Next, there was a change in her personality and she became extremely demanding and stubborn. Ten minutes later she had calmed down. Chlorine had triggered a hyperactive state, silliness, and personality change. She was exposed to chlorine *every day* in her drinking water, as well as to chlorine-containing scouring powder and laundry bleach.

Mixed tree pollens: Laura did not get the usual pollen reactions of sneezing, nasal discharge, red eyes, or itching of the ears and throat, that allergists expect in cases of pollen allergy. Instead of hay fever symptoms, she had itching of her arms and legs, and her face became flushed. Itching and flushing indicated that something in the tree pollen extract was being absorbed and was producing symptoms in her body far from the usual hay fever sites. There were no visible changes in the skin of her arms and legs where the itching was localized. It is probable that there were changes in the circulation deep within her head and along with the flushing there also might have been changes in her brain. She had no mental symptoms, but since doctors do not know why it is we "itch" in the first place, it is possible that the pollen stirred up some nervous system mechanism that resulted in the sensation of itching in her skin.

Baker's yeast: No reaction. This is a very common offender, and this test also served as a control test.

Food preservative mixture: Laura sneezed vigorously and developed a nose bleed. Allergic nose bleeds are very common in children. Allergy has been established as the major cause of this frequent problem in childhood.*

All-purpose spray (for vegetable gardens, flowers, trees and shrubs): She became very angry and irritable and was unable to get along with any of the other children being tested. Then she developed generalized itching, became very quiet and moderately tired. She went from a hyper state to a hypo state like a minor manic-depressive reaction. Foods she was eating every day contained residues of spray material, and sprays were used in her general area on shrubs, flowers, and trees, as well as on vegetable gardens. Exposure to this insect spray was an important factor in her emotional-behavioral problems, itching, and fatigue.

---

*Dr. Hosen went to a supermarket and spent several hours reading labels and listing all of the substances that were added to various foods. With the assistance of his brother-in-law, a chemist, Dr. Hosen obtained thirteen of the preservatives listed on the packages of food. In order to economize for patients, instead of testing each substance individually, we mixed them together. Dr. Hosen's combination of thirteen commonly used preservatives has been used by both of us in thousands of tests. He and I have both been able to demonstrate that these materials are important factors in physical and mental disturbances.

Comment: In performing tests with various chemical agents, I start with one or two drops of a very weak solution of the testing materials and then employ progressively stronger doses, each test solution being five times as strong as the previous one. Tests are continued until there is a sufficient reaction to demonstrate the presence of bio-ecologic illness, and at this point it is stopped. The strongest dose I use of various weed killers (herbicides), fruit tree sprays, or vegetable garden sprays is usually one-fifth of the regular strength recommended by the manufacturer as the safe concentration to apply to flowers or vegetables. These solutions are handled by home gardeners who are exposed to them when they mix them, when they spray them, and when they eat the garden and orchard products that have received this spraying. The test solution only $\frac{1}{25}$ as strong as the regularly used spray caused an episode of negative behavior, and Laura could not get along with other children in the room. With a solution one-fifth as strong as the regular spray, she had itching of her neck and elbows. Theregular-strength material made her very quiet. This series of graduated doses of garden spray reproduced many of her usual symptoms.

Bacterial vaccine: Laura had itching of the lower back, hips, and upper thighs. She did not respond when she was addressed by the technicians, and she didn't seem to hear during the test.

Comment: I use a mixture of many respiratory vaccines prepared from bacteria that are normally present in the respiratory tract and from those that cause respiratory infections, including "cold" germs, strep germs, staph germs, pneumonia germs, etc. This test shows allergic sensitivity to respiratory bacteria, and suggests that there may be a tendency to develop respiratory infections.

Fruit tree spray: Generalized itching of the skin and deep within her ears, associated with vaginal and anal itching.

Comment: I have seen many patients with no visible rash or inflammation of the genitals or anus who were told there was nothing wrong after they had been examined for bacterial or yeast (monilia) infection and tested several times for pinworms. Doctors find nothing and so the patients are told that their problems are psychosomatic.

Cigarette tobacco: She became hyperactive.

Yellow food coloring (FD&C #5, tartrazine): She became moderately tired with her first dose and had slight itching.

Comment: Yellow #5 is widely used (when mixed with red, it makes an orange color). Yellow dye is used in medications, candy, desserts, soda; it is added to the vinegar in pickles to make a uniform color. Often bakers put it in cakes and cookies when they want to make their customers think that their products were made with egg yolks or a rich dough.

Each food color is a different substance chemically and it is possible for a person to react to one food color and not another or to have a different reaction to each of them. It is possible that a person sensitive to one color would develop sensitivity to other food colors (and synthetic flavors) if there was a heavy exposure to them. Heavy exposure is not uncommon because a person could be eating an artificially colored and flavored gelatin dessert often, and be drinking large quantities of artificially colored and flavored sodas. This problem can be compounded by the fact that there are often preservatives in soda as well as corn sugar and cane sugar. It is possible for an individual to be simultaneously exposed to many foods that are combined in a "disaster mixture."

The United States government certifies "pure" food colors; what is certified is that they are coal-tar derived colors that meet certain specifications. This does not mean that people will not have reactions after ingesting them, because a government certification does not consider their biologic activity as allergic excitants. Recent emphasis on the importance of food coloring and synthetic flavors in hyperactivity by Dr. Benjamin Feingold (whose work I have already discussed) may give people an incorrect impression that these artificial colors and flavors cause only hyperactivity and not other adverse effects. I have shown that each food color can produce different symptoms in different people, and this definitely includes adults. One person will get a headache; another will have asthma. Someone else may have abdominal discomfort or joint pains or itching or become restless or depressed. One of my pediatric patients had a bladder reaction with painful urination from red lollypops, but other colored lollypops were well tolerated.

Alternaria (mold): Her handwriting became very untidy. Her throat and vagina itched. She developed abdominal pains like gas pains.

Comment: Here is a little girl, plagued by genital itching not due to pinworms, who might frequently scratch and rub herself to relieve an allergic itch. This itching (with an organic basis), which caused genital manipulation, could easily be misinterpreted because she appeared to be masturbating. Allergic reactions in the genital and anal area occur quite frequently and are often responsible for a great deal of discomfort in members of both sexes. A number of gynecologists have informed me that they are often puzzled by patients who complain of severe vaginal and anal itching in whom they can find no evidence of a physical disorder other than some scratch marks or local irritation secondary to vigorous scratching. In the absence of any form of infection, they usually conclude that the patient has an emotional problem: a neurotic anxiety conditioned by her attitude toward sexual activities, or as a form of hostility or resentment toward her mate. The correct diagnosis and appropriate management of such cases is usually not a difficult problem for me to solve, and with each success, months or years of discomfort and worry are wiped away.

Fusarium (mold): Laura acted very silly and became extremely active. She was unable to sit still and jumped around the room. She kept humming in a high-pitched voice. Her mother said, "We came here for this type of reaction. This happens a lot."

Pullularia (mold): Laura became slightly hyper with the first dose and with the second dose her hyperactivity increased: She became very "snippy" and fresh. She hummed in a high-pitched voice, another test-induced flare-up characteristic of her typical behavior problems.

Hormodendrum (mold): Laura did not react to this very common mold.

   Comment: Some allergists who are not aware of the importance of other species of mold limit their attention to alternaria and hormodendrum. Hormodendrum is an important mold but if an individual does not react to it or to alternaria, my studies have shown that an allergist cannot conclude that the patient is not sensitive to any other molds. Many allergists make the error of limiting their mold testing to hormodendrum and alternaria and assume that they have adequately examined the patient for mold sensitivity. Although Laura did not react to hormodendrum, important symptoms were provoked by aspergillus, fusarium, pullularia, monilia, and penicillium. Mold testing must be comprehensive.

Monilia (mold): Laura became extremely hyperactive and hopped about the room on one foot. She refused to give us a handwriting sample. She was cranky, irritable, and unwilling to share her toys. Next, she was on the verge of tears, and soon thereafter she became depressed.

Comment: Monilia is a yeastlike organism closely related to molds and it causes many symptoms. Vaginal and rectal itching often occur after an individual has taken an antibiotic that kills intestinal bacteria and permits monilia to grow unchecked due to the absence of the bacteria that were eliminated. This is why many physicians advise patients to take buttermilk, acidophilus milk, or yogurt to replace the bacteria that have been eliminated by an antibiotic.

Penicillium (mold): The area beneath her eyes turned red, and Laura had sharp pains in her upper teeth. Then, as had been noted at home and in school, she became incapable of understanding the content of a conversation—she did not know what the people around her were saying.

Comment: On a number of occasions I have observed toothache as an allergic symptom induced by testing. It is important for dentists to know that allergy can cause pain in an otherwise normal tooth.

After testing was concluded, we launched an intensive campaign to clean up Laura's home environment. Her diet was arranged to avoid foods that caused moderate to severe reactions; test-negative and mild-reacting foods were incorporated in a Rotary Diversified Diet.

The house had to be thoroughly cleaned in an allergic sense from top to bottom by dusting, vacuuming, and scrubbing. We did our best to eliminate all forms of chemical air pollutants within the home; this included petroleum-derived substances and chlorine-containing materials. All of these substances have been mentioned elsewhere so I only mention a few of them here, such as waxes, polishes, air fresheners, hair sprays, detergents, disinfectants, window cleaners, oven cleaners, laundry bleach, perfume, cosmetics, etc. Smoking was prohibited. The gas stove was removed. The car had to be parked in a location where fumes would not enter the house. Odorous plastics or rubber goods were removed. No paint, paintbrushes, or varnishes could be stored in the house. Everything that bothered her had to go immediately if Laura was to have an opportunity to become and remain well.

The measures I recommended for Laura's family to follow involved some expenses, considerable effort, and careful attention to many details. Yet, no reasonable measure could ever be considered "too much." Laura's IQ of 120 and her abilities were being wasted a good part of the time. What was at stake here was the continued normal functioning of a child's developing brain—happiness, intellectual achievement, productivity, and relationships with all the other people involved in her life.

We must be comprehensive in the environmental controls and dietary programs we initiate. At times, radical changes are required of an individual and his family. But if the measures are inconvenient or seem to be expensive when they are initiated, the illness must be seen in perspective. By establishing and following a comprehensive program of bio-ecologic management, we may be avoiding years of costly special education as well as psychiatric care in and out of hospitals that would have to be paid for by the family or the taxpayers. There are goals that will never be achieved, intellectual satisfaction that will never be realized, a sense of personal achievement that will never be felt, if the patient with a reversible form of bio-ecologic illness remains untreated and continues to suffer from this disorder.

In September of 1977, we contacted Laura's mother to see how Laura was progressing. Her report was gratifying. It was evident that Laura was on the road to recovery. Her teacher had written that "Laura was able to complete her work and she seems more content."

CASE STUDY: CHILDHOOD SCHIZOPHRENIA/DEAFNESS/MOTOR DIFFICULTIES/FATIGUE

Jonny Y.'s mother suffered from toxemia of pregnancy, and when he was born in the intensive care unit of his local hospital, it was evident that he had been affected by his mother's illness:

He was very small, his color was "bloody-gray," and he was quiet and sleepy.

From the beginning, his development was abnormal. He didn't even open his eyes or cry for the first six weeks of his life, and when his mother introduced milk formulas to his diet they were usually rejected by violent "projectile" vomiting. For the first two years of his life, he had almost constant diarrhea.

He had poor head control at a time when other children his age were able to look around easily, and he sat up much later than his peers. He still was crawling when other children his age were walking well, and when he attempted to speak at a normal age, he had great difficulty putting phrases together and often his pronunciation was unclear. When he got a little older, he also began to experience hallucinations—voices coming out of nowhere. Then he began to have two-week periods of normal behavior, which would be followed by four-week periods of difficult behavior during which he would be quiet and subdued one moment and screaming in fear and impossible to control the next.

Because he had difficulty speaking, his parents' early impression was that Jonny was unable to understand language rather than to use speech. They felt his problem was based on a hearing problem because there were occasions when they had to scream at him to get a response, although at other times they had only to speak in a normal voice and he would react. His parents also noticed that these fluctuations in his ability to hear seemed somehow to be related to the time of the year.

His slow progress, suspected hearing problem, language difficulty, and behavioral problems led to a series of studies at Johns Hopkins Hospital, the world-famous institution in Baltimore, Maryland, where the doctors found that Jonny's parents were correct—he had a 40 percent hearing loss in his right ear and a 60 percent hearing loss in his left ear; at Johns Hopkins they also diagnosed his personality problems and hallucinations as childhood schizophrenia.

When his parents brought him into my consultation room, the first thing I noticed was his rubbing his nose from side to side with his index finger, giving me a typical "allergic salute"

—practically a guarantee that I am looking at an allergic child. When his mother told me about the projectile vomiting associated with his early formula, this suggested the possibility that he may have had a severe gastrointestinal allergy to something in the formula. The fact that his loss of hearing fluctuated from time to time indicated that his hearing difficulty might very well be a recurring allergic problem of variable intensity rather than a form of permanent damage that a constant level of deafness would indicate.

In reviewing his dietary history, I found he had gone off on occasional food binges with crackers, candy, or potato chips, which suggested that wheat, yeast, milk, vanilla, chocolate, corn sugar, or potato might be allergies of the addictive kind.

I became increasingly suspicious of food allergies when Mrs. Y. recalled that on Valentine's Day Jonny had eaten a rather large quantity of red candy and five hours later had suffered severe abdominal cramps, diarrhea, and vomiting. (At the time his mother did not associate his gastrointestinal illness with the red candies. Instead, she thought that Jonny had a "stomach virus," although no one else in the family became ill.) He was sick all the next day with the same symptoms when, suddenly and dramatically, he placed his hands over his ears and screamed in fear for someone to please tell the "voices" to stop ordering him to eat more candy.

I suspected that his unusual behavior was a withdrawal reaction from some food or chemical in the red candy that might have first caused him to have the acute symptoms of vomiting, diarrhea, and abdominal cramps and then caused him to experience an addictive craving for the red candy and a hallucination that "voices" were ordering him to eat it.

Jonny's mother also told me that he usually had pain in his left eye and left forehead and often complained of severe pressure behind his left eye. In addition, he had chronic fatigue* and was

*Chronic fatigue in both adults and children is a complaint that doctors encounter many times a day in every field of medicine. Many patients have told me that they can sleep for eight to twelve hours a night, and when they wake up in the morning they still are not the least bit refreshed. Some have stated that they feel they might as well not have gone to bed for all the good that sleeping did them. I have found that allergy and allergic withdrawal are at the

not refreshed in the morning despite eight to ten hours of sleep each night. Whether he had adequate sleep or not, he was usually irritable in the morning, and at the end of the school day, his mother "never knew exactly what to expect when he came through the door." On some days he would be charming and pleasant after school; on other days he would be a "monster" who screamed and cursed at her.

When I reviewed Jonny's chemical history with him, he stated that he could not stand it when his mother smoked. It made him cough and sneeze and feel as if he could not breathe. His eyes would burn and become red. In addition, many odors, he added, made him sick. He said he could not name all of them, but nail polish and his mother's hair spray made him nauseous. (If his teacher polished her nails in class, it would make him literally gag.) Exhaust fumes from cars and trucks made him extremely uncomfortable in a nonspecific fashion; all he could say was "I can't stand them." Sometimes the chlorinated water supply in the house made him feel tired, confused, and depressed. If Jonny's mother used bleach in the laundry or cleaned the sink or tub with a scouring powder containing chlorine, he would promptly detect the presence of chlorine there too and become ill. He told me that he thought he would be poisoned by chlorine someday because it was so "bad" for him. Keep in mind that this is a child who had been diagnosed as having a severe form of illness—schizophrenia! Like many of my patients, Jonny told me that he could not say exactly how many substances affected him but he was very much aware of the fact that he didn't "feel right" after an exposure to them, and, therefore, did not like them. These complaints are not nebulous; they are symptoms of an allergy just a hair's breadth below the level of awareness.

As much as Johnny hated the smell of chlorine, he loved the odor of gasoline and permanent marking pens and felt he got

---

root of almost every chronic fatigue complaint I have ever seen. What happens is that the person suffering from chronic fatigue is unconscious, and to all outward appearances is sleeping quietly, but because of allergies, he begins to experience delayed withdrawal reactions that persist throughout the night. Therefore, although he is unconscious, his sleep is not truly restful, and in the morning the night's rest has not been of any benefit whatsoever.

a lift from them. Disliking or hating certain things, liking or loving other things is the result of having an allergy to them. Actually, the petrochemical substances he encountered all day long made him feel below par (his allergic reaction), and a quick sniff of the volatile agents present in gasoline or a marking pen was just enough to make him feel better (stop his allergic addictive withdrawal reaction.)

Jonny frequently had athlete's foot infections, which indicated that he was susceptible to certain species of mold. His mother said that he had itched and scratched all of his life for "no apparent reason." Allergic itching is very common and is often caused by mold sensitivity. This made the construction of his family's house important, because it was built on a concrete slab without a basement or crawl space and, therefore, the main floor was in direct contact with the ground. In summertime, when the ground under the house was cooler than the surrounding air, the slab floor also was cool; there would be condensation of moisture under the carpet, and mold would begin to grow. The house was also filled with potted plants, from which the odor of mildew was quite obvious to the entire family.

Jonny would become hyperactive immediately after breakfast every weekday. However, he was all right on weekends. When I investigated his diet, I found he was having more milk on weekdays at school than he normally drank at home on weekends. He also ate eggs every morning prior to leaving for school, but on weekends his mother always prepared pancakes for him, made without any eggs.

I tested Jonny extensively because of the seriousness of his problems. It was significant that there were a number of negative tests in various categories of common environmental substances which served as controls. A number of the major offending foods that cause serious problems in many other patients did not affect him at all. A number of the foods he was currently eating did not produce any reactions. He selectively reacted to some molds but not to others, to some of the chemical tests and not others. He even reacted to the toothpaste he had been using. This is what testing for allergies revealed:

Cane sugar: Slightly tired, slightly dizzy, and a mild headache. He coughed a few times. He felt "funny," but he was not able to tell exactly how he felt or where he felt funny.

Milk: Itching of his left eye and a dull headache in the left temple. Coughing. He acted very silly and giddy. He said it felt as though something was pushing his left eye forward and out of his head. Then, he became detached from his surroundings and said, "I feel like I am not here. My spirit is leaving my body."

Wheat: Headache. Eyes burning. Sleepy. Dizzy. His cheeks became very pale. His mother stated that facial pallor was something that they saw very often, and it would come and go.

Eggs: Throat itching. Mild cough. Mild headache. Eyes hurt.

Beef: Coughing. Dizziness. Feeling of being separated from surroundings. Headache coming and going throughout this test.

Peanut (which he loved dearly in the form of peanut butter): Severe headache across forehead and left side of his head. According to his mother, who was present throughout all of the testing, he acted very "goofy, silly, and giddy." Coughing.

Banana: Silly. Talkative. Giggly. Dizzy.

Tomato: Drowsy. Headache above eyes.

Tree pollen: Sneezing. Mild headache. Became silly.

Grass pollens: Swelling of his left eyelid, which became half closed.

Saccharin (the sweetener in his favorite diet drinks): Weak, shaky. Said his legs felt "nervous." Dizzy. Tense.

Weed pollens: Feet felt tingly and as though they were "falling asleep." He got up and walked around the room. Became very tired and drowsy.

Lettuce: He felt that he wasn't getting enough air into his lungs, and his heart was pounding.

Apple: Hyperactive. Whistling. He pretended he was blowing a musical instrument. Silly. Making faces, talking loudly. Then he developed a headache in his forehead, became drowsy, and slowed down. His mother described this reaction as "a real wild one."

Cola: His ears swelled up and turned bright red. His ears usually were generally swollen, with the lobes more so, especially the left ear. With this test, they became inflamed looking and very swollen. His face and eyelids became puffy, his face red and blotchy.

Maltox (all-purpose estate spray): Both ears became moderately swol-

Usual
Handwriting

Beginning of
House Dust
Reaction

Becoming
Hyperactive

Becoming
Listless,
Depressed

len and red. His eyes itched. There was pressure in the right side of his head.

House dust: Argumentative. Annoyed. Then he became angry and crabby. He cried. He ran down the hall and rushed off and locked himself in the bathroom so he wouldn't be bothered by anyone. When he came out, he was very quiet.

Yellow food coloring: As he became aware of the early stages of this reaction, he said "Here it comes again!" He became hyperactive, threw himself down on the floor, and became giddy and loud. Then he ran down the hall and hit his mother. He was given a neutralizing dose and calmed down quickly.*

Toothpaste (brand name withheld): Dull, temporal headache that gradually extended from his left temple around to the forehead.

---

*This test with FD&C Yellow #5 (tartrazine) is further evidence to support Dr. Benjamin Feingold's work regarding food coloring as an important cause of hyperactivity in children. But please look at Jonny's reactions to milk, peanut, banana, tree pollens, dust, and apple for additional evidence that hyperactivity is a cerebral dysfunction from *many* causes.

Jonny was a child with a long, difficult past who, in addition to motor problems and hearing loss, had serious allergic manifestations that I feel explained at least some of his mental, emotional, perceptual, and behavioral problems. The bio-ecologic illness that caused his ears to swell may even be related to internal changes that could cause his fluctuating loss of hearing. Naturally, a child who doesn't hear well to begin with is going to be unhappy and difficult to manage. Obviously, modern medicine desperately needs a comprehensive approach to serious problems such as this one, which goes far beyond my present knowledge and skills.

Babies and Formula(s)

The first fact that I wish to emphasize is that no milk can possibly be better for a baby than milk from its own species. A mother's breast provides a necessary premilk substance, colostrum, which may be crucial for the early health of the baby because it gives greater resistance to infection. Human milk is a complete and perfect food specifically designed to satisfy the needs of an infant. Even though many babies will be able to tolerate various foods at an early age, a baby's gastrointestinal tract and physiology were really designed for him to be fed milk exclusively for the first year or two of his life. Although the cow has been honored with the title of "foster mother of the human race" and has performed this service with considerable distinction, mother nature intended cow's milk for the nutrition of calves in the same way that goat's milk is designed for kids and ewe's milk is nature's specific food for early nutrition of lambs.

In a series of food tests of allergic infants, 50 percent were found to be allergic to milk and 48 percent were found to be allergic to corn.* Since most formulas with an evaporated-milk base contain cow's milk and corn, you can see why many babies react to them. If an evaporated-milk formula does not contain corn, it may have cane sugar or some other carbohydrate. For-

*Tennie Mae Lunceford, "The Clinical Management of Infant Allergy." *Clinical Ecology*, L. Dickey, ed. (Springfield, Ill.: Charles C. Thomas, 1976), p. 645.

mulas made with a soybean base, with the exception of Mull-soy, contain corn. (In addition, you have to be alerted for possible allergies to coconut oil and maltose or other food products that are present in some formulas.) The only meat-base formula that does not contain corn is Gerber's Meat Base®, which contains sesame oil and tapioca, and they may cause problems if a child is sensitive to them. The lamb formula does contain corn.

Any baby who reacts to a particular formula, whether it is after a few days or after having taken fifty or five hundred bottles of the formula, is probably allergic to one or more of the ingredients in it. (At times there are other reasons, but food intolerance must always be ruled out unless the reason is obvious—illness, very rapid feeding, formula too cold, baby frightened or upset, etc.) Reactive babies have a hereditary predisposition to allergies that was passed on to them by either their mother or their father. The course of their allergic predisposition can take one of two directions: they can become sensitized to particular foods while they are *in the womb* because their mother repeatedly eats the same foods over and over again. In this case, when they encounter one of the foods to which they are now actively allergic in their first bottle of formula, they react. The second direction a predisposition toward allergies can take is that the baby can be born with his predisposition there, but dormant. If this is the case, then it takes either a few bottles of formula or a great many bottles, depending on the strength of the predisposition, to trigger an allergic response.

How to Treat an Allergic Baby

The solution? You should never feed your baby the same food more than once in four or five days. *Never* give him a food from the same biologic family of foods on consecutive days. This principle is called "rotation."

The best way to approach formula feeding by rotation is to take four or five totally *different* formulas and rotate them by feeding one formula for one twenty-four-hour period and another formula for the next twenty-four-hour period, etc. At the end of four or five days, return to the first formula, and begin the series again. If your baby reacts to one of the formulas, eliminate it and substitute a totally different formula. *Always rotate.* This may help baby tolerate foods in the formula to which he is mildly or moderately allergic by eliminating overexposure to them and will make the appearance of new food allergy much less likely. Of course, some babies are allergic to some ingredient(s) in every commercially prepared formula. If this should be so with your baby, you can take meats, fruit, and vegetables, puree them, mix them with warm spring water, and find out which foods your baby can tolerate. *It is important, however, to remember that frequent exposure to foods from the same family can ultimately create an allergy to members of that food family.* Therefore, at least two to three days should pass before the baby is given a food from the same family.

Test for Infants of Any Age

If your baby cannot tolerate any formulas or if you would like to test him for allergic physical and mental symptoms that may be associated with foods, the following 5-Day Preliminary Test is recommended.

INSTRUCTIONS

Begin environmental controls as discussed in chapter 6.

Separate the test meals by at least three to four hours. Gradually increase the amount given.

Between feedings give your baby warm spring water.

Puree everything not already liquid. Add spring water to juices.

It is preferable to use organically grown food in order to eliminate pesticides, insecticides, herbicides, food coloring, preservatives, etc.

Puree raw fruits and lightly cooked vegetables with as little water as possible so that the nutrients remain. Do not add salt or sugar.

Write down baby's reactions every ten minutes for the first hour after a test meal.

In order to make this test diet as useful as possible for many people, there are several test meals in which you may make a choice of the foods you wish to use. As long as a food is eaten once on the day that it is scheduled for, it does not matter which time of day it is eaten. For example, on Day #1, rice could be taken in the morning and apple could be taken as Meal #4 in the evening; on Day #2 chicken could be taken as Meal #2 and lima bean could be taken as Meal #3, etc. If your baby has been hospitalized for convulsions, severe asthma—any life threatening ailment—do *not* perform this test without the careful supervision of a qualified bio-ecologic physician.

	MEAL #1	MEAL #2	MEAL #3	MEAL #4
Day #1	Apple	Squash or pumpkin	Lamb or scallops	Rice or beet
Day #2	Apricot	Lima bean	Chicken	Buckwheat or turnip
Day #3	Pear	Carrot	Pork	Cod or haddock
Day #4	Peach or cantaloupe	Sweet potato	Turkey	Oat
Day #5	Banana	White potato	Sole or flounder	Pea or string bean

AFTER THE TEST DIET

At the conclusion of the testing period, you will have a list of foods that your baby tolerated, and another list of foods to which he is allergic. Now go to chapter 9 to get instructions on testing *all* the foods. Keep in mind that caloric requirements are determined on the basis of body measurements but the final criteria for meeting a child's needs depend upon the growth pattern and the sense of well-being.

Caloric requirements are 50 calories per pound during infancy, 45 calories per pound from age one to three, 41 calories per pound from four to six, 36 calories per pound from seven to nine, 32 calories per pound from ten to twelve. The average distribution of calories in a well-balanced diet is as follows: protein 15 percent, fat 35 percent and carbohydrates 50 percent.

In general, a consistent caloric imbalance of 500 calories per day will result in a body weight change of about one pound per week.

How to Test School-Age Children for Food Allergy

Testing infants does not usually present a problem since they do not have any control over their diet. However, it may be difficult to have a schoolchild follow his preliminary diet when he is away from home. Even if you prepare lunch for your child to take to school, there can be problems with food swapping with classmates. Or a child may purchase snacks or soda from a dispensing machine or obtain a dessert in the cafeteria or share a snack with a friend. In addition, if food addiction is an important part of your child's problem, cravings for specific foods may be very difficult for a child to handle, and it is best to begin a rotary diet during a vacation period. If the nature of the disorder is serious enough to warrant it, a child can benefit by being kept out of school until the preliminary diet is well completed and foods he is not allergic to are established. No child should be kept out of school unless there is an excellent reason for doing so, but if the child's behavior or academic performance can be benefited, it is more important to initiate a diet than to send a troubled or uncomfortable child to school.

Considerable improvement and, at times, amazing results may be seen after just five days on a simple rotary test diet. During or after the child's test, you may find it helpful to enlist the aid of various individuals in the school. Explain what you are doing and why you are doing it. You may be surprised by the enthusiastic cooperation that some teachers and teacher's aides and school officials will give you once they understand your objectives. This cooperation may extend far beyond the supervision of a child's eating; in a most favorable situation, the teachers and other school personnel may make some very useful observations regarding your child's behavior and performance at various times of the day. This would give you valuable information concerning the possible effects of breakfast and lunch. At the same time, we must not ignore any environmental factors related to classroom activities and possible chemical exposures that may occur because of various maintenance procedures or other activities in nearby classrooms or shops. Don't forget that trips to the bathroom or the front office may be associated with exposure to disinfectant and deodorizing chemicals, or duplicating fluids and glues and other office supplies.

HOW TO BEGIN

There are two ways for a child to begin the rotary diet. The first is to fast on spring water from glass jars for at least five days. At the end of five days, the intestinal tract is cleared of food residues, and the child is in a hyper-reactive state so that food reactions may be dramatic and leave no doubt in the mind of parent or child that the child is allergic. Besides, after a five-day fast, the child usually feels terrific.

If a child is not too thin, five days without food will not make him lose much weight. Since it takes a lack of about 500 calories a day for one week to lose a pound, the most he probably will lose (unless some of his weight is due to retained fluid) is two or three pounds. And it is very much worth trying when the possible benefits are realized.

The first few days of a fast, the child may be mildly to moderately uncomfortable. (I fasted six days myself with no ill effects other than fatigue and a mild headache.) Hunger usually ceases very quickly after the first day, and any discomfort, physical or mental, or cravings for specific foods thereafter are usually the result of going through withdrawal from the foods to which the fasting person has an addictive allergy. If the child is uncomfortable during the first few days of fasting, it's a sign that he is freeing his system of a chronic addictive burden. On the morning of the sixth day, after five days of fasting on spring water, give him his first food test. Write down the date, day, time, and name of the food, and record pulse changes and any symptoms; describe the reaction in detail.

The second way to approach a test diet is to have the child avoid all the foods that appear in the test diet for five days prior to beginning the test. Although I recommend the fast, if your child cannot fast then this second method must be used. It is not as reliable an approach to testing because hidden foods are difficult to avoid; also, the child may be responding allergically to foods other than those that appear in the preliminary test diet. If you opt for food elimination rather than fasting, you must scrupulously read all package labels—and when in doubt as to all the ingredients in a food mix, do not let the child eat it.

MAKING YOUR CHILD BETTER MAY INVOLVE MAKING HIM WORSE INITIALLY

Many children can be tested at home for food and environmental allergy. The steps are simple to take. But I must emphasize, as the case histories indicated, that the results during the fasting or food elimination period, and during the tests themselves can temporarily exacerbate the problems under investigation. A child may have chronic fatigue that is caused by bananas, wheat, and pork. When he is tested at home for allergy to these foods, he is probably going to experience his familiar fatigue symptoms, but possibly to a much greater degree than ususal. The child who has trouble getting up in the morning may seem exhausted and fall sound asleep minutes after he eats bananas or wheat or pork. The child who has mental confusion, hyperactivity, headache, and itching as symptoms could become disoriented, stuporous, or overactive and develop a severe itching. I do not want to frighten any parents, but I want to warn them that if a child's symptoms include severe asthma, epilepsy, or uncontrollable destructive behavior that can be life-or property-threatening, the child should be tested under the supervision of a qualified bio-ecologic physician—not at home by parents. For the most part, parents who want to test their children without the above severe problems should be able to put the child on a rotary diet; some will observe fantastic results.

I have children give me writing samples as they are being

tested. Changes in penmanship are a concrete evidence that the brain is being affected by a food or chemical test. I have children read as they are being tested. A number of children suddenly become unable to concentrate and to comprehend what they are reading, or they may forget what they have just read by the time they reach the end of a sentence. It is not unusual for visual blurring to develop or to have words misread or to have slower speech or stuttering.

5-DAY PRELIMINARY TEST DIET FOR PRE-SCHOOLERS AND SCHOOL-AGE CHILDREN

Begin environmental controls as outlined in chapter 6. Fast or avoid all foods for five days before starting this test. See Appendix for detailed instructions. Then begin with Day #1. Note that these foods are exactly the same as the "Test Diet for Infants"; preparation of food differs, however.

	MEAL #1	MEAL #2	MEAL #3	MEAL #4
Day #1	Apple	Squash or pumpkin	Lamb or scallops	Rice or beet
Day #2	Apricot	Lima bean	Chicken	Buckwheat or turnip
Day #3	Pear	Carrot	Pork	Cod or haddock
Day #4	Peach or cantaloupe	Sweet potato	Turkey	Oat
Day #5	Banana	White potato	Sole or flounder	Pea or string bean

AFTER THE TEST

Your child has now tested at least twenty foods, but there are many more foods left to test. Turn to chapter 9, and continue testing.

A Special Plea to Teachers

When I think of the numbers of allergic children with whom teachers have to deal every day—children whose symptoms include hyperactivity, irritability, "goofy" behavior, violence, fatigue, restlessness, and just about any other mental disturbance you can name—I think of the terrible mistakes that many well-intentioned, fine teachers make when they try to discipline or control these children.

Every child who has entered my office with what I call "cerebral" allergy has been a child who, when not reacting, wanted to please, wanted to do well, wanted to be accepted. Eccentric behavior in class is not necessarily a deliberate, self-destructive course of action, but it may well be that the nervous system is totally incapable of functioning normally because it is under allergic distress. The child who reads well once in a while and poorly other times; the child whose handwriting is poor one day and fine the next; the child who can sit still in the morning, but is impossible to control in the afternoon—each of these children may be demonstrating cerebral allergy.

One young girl's mother related the story of how her child had been sitting in art class about half done with a really artistic poster when the teacher came over and complimented the child on her good work. Two minutes later, when the teacher glanced back at the child, the little girl was scrawling all over her work. It seemed to the teacher as though the child were willfully destroying the poster because the teacher had paid her a compliment. This teacher was a fine woman who loved teaching and whose students liked her; but even one dedicated to her work and to her students can totally misinterpret the actions of an allergic child in the throes of a reaction. The child's teacher felt this was a stubborn, antagonistic, antisocial act and the child's way of asserting herself. But when I spoke to the child, she did not know what she had done. She said, "It just happened." When I tested this child, it turned out she was highly allergic to petroleum byproducts. The permanent marker ink had toluene derived from petroleum. She inhaled the toluene fumes, and they triggered her seemingly willful behavior.

Without knowledge of allergy and the dramatic effect it can have on a child's behavior, often the classroom becomes a battlefield where the allergic student and his teacher are engaged in a conflict that neither can win.

6
Environmental Allergies

Question: When you leave your apartment or house, do you begin to feel better? If you leave for a week-long trip, do you find your head clears, your migraine disappears, dizziness stops, your aches and pains subside, depression fades away, and your entire attitude is better? If so, chemical pollution of the atmosphere in your home may be making you ill.

It may come as a surprise to you to discover just how badly polluted the air in your home is. Last year, scientists from the Lawrence Berkeley Laboratory told a clean-air congress in Tokyo that the level of air pollution in a home is often higher and more dangerous than that outside the home. This conclusion was based on an analysis of six homes in the Berkeley, California, area. Hand-held monitors were used to measure the levels of commonly found pollutants. The researchers found that the major sources of pollutants were the heating systems, gas stoves, fumes from cooking, and cigarette smoke.

Even if the homeowners had turned on exhaust fans while using a gas oven for cooking, it took only one hour at 350° to produce concentrations of carbon monoxide and nitrogen dioxide that were the equivalent of the notorious Los Angeles smog that we constantly read and hear about. If the kitchen fan was not turned on while the oven was at 350°, the concentrations of these two potent chemicals soared to levels that were three times as great! When the study moved from the kitchen into the bedroom, it was found that gas-fired central heating was capable of polluting the air with nitrogen dioxide and nitric oxide to a level that was three times as high as that recommended by the federal air-quality standards.

The level of air pollution in the home can also be greatly increased by fumes from detergents and disinfectants jammed under the kitchen sink; from the hair sprays, under-arm deodorants, colognes, air fresheners, nail polishes, and nail polish removers on the shelf behind the bathroom mirror; from the furniture and floor waxes and polishes, the moth flakes and insect sprays, the paints, turpentines, varnishes, and so forth in the utility closet. The containers and dispensers may look airtight when they are recapped, but they usually leak; and when the tops are removed, the process of contamination begins in full force. Many of these product labels actually read: "Use in a well-ventilated room. Avoid prolonged contact. Do not inhale or swallow. Keep out of the reach of children. Call physician immediately."

The residues from the chemicals used to give each brand of cigarette its own distinctive flavor and aroma, from the highly poisonous insecticide sprays applied to the tobacco crop as it was growing, and from the kerosene heating unit used to keep the tobacco warm while it was being cured in a barn all remain in the cigarette—none of the residues are removed. So in homes where there is smoking, the smoker and those in the same room with him are inhaling the burning fumes of extremely toxic agents which are accepted as a normal part of tobacco agricultural technology, as well as the particles of tobacco and the actual tobacco smoke.

What is especially ironic about cigarette smoke is that while the smoker is addicted to the chemicals and/or the tobacco in the cigarette, and is having his or her own problems, the nonsmokers in the house can be desperately allergic to the cigarette, pipe, or cigar tobacco or the chemical fumes generated when it is burned or smoked. If their eyes don't immediately get red or they don't instantly have trouble breathing, they may become depressed or develop a migraine headache a few hours later, but no one ever suspects that smoking is a major factor in these serious health problems affecting nonsmoking members of the family.

The final clincher to chemical air pollution permeating the

house can come from a garage built right under a bedroom, or next to and opening into the kitchen, den, family room, or playroom. The fumes from the exhaust spewing out of the car when it is started in the morning, or for those few minutes when the engine is still running after the car has been brought back into the garage can cause incredible allergic problems for the family members who are chemically sensitive to petrochemicals and petroleum byproducts. In the morning the fumes seep up into the house as the car is backed out of the garage and down the driveway. If the garage door is then shut, if those fumes have not had a chance to escape, part of them have many hours in which to slip through the house. At night, as the car sits in the garage, not only do residual exhaust fumes hover in the air, but fumes from the carburetor, the gas tank, oil leaks, and the car lubricants join the exhaust. Throw in a workbench and shelves laden with oils, car waxes, paints, and glues, plus gasoline; add a lawn mower to the corner of the garage, and you have all the necessary ingredients for a huge allergic chemical reaction in a family member who may be sleeping over the garage or sitting in an adjoining room.

CASE STUDY: CLAUSTROPHOBIA/FATIGUE/ANXIETY/DEPRESSION/PAINFUL MENSTRUATION AND INTERCOURSE

A twenty-five-year-old married woman came into my office complaining of chronic nasal symptoms, hives, and frequent episodes of laryngitis. Her menstruation was always extremely uncomfortable; she suffered from fatigue, anxiety, and depression. Hers was the kind of case that had not responded fully to medical treatment, and it had been easy for other doctors to diagnose some of her problems as allergies and some, whose cause could not be determined, as either emotional or mental (psychosomatic) because *everyone* knows that anxiety and depression are "mental" disorders.

She came from an emotionally turbulent home. Her mother was "emotionally intense," and, she said, her father was "incapacitated by miner's asthma, excitable, wild-tempered, and frightening." She had much resentment against an older brother who was "Mother's favorite." A younger brother was a "wild drinker" and had had several car accidents.

At the age of twenty-three she had had a laparotomy (an exploratory abdominal operation) to determine if there was any abnormal internal disorder within her abdomen or pelvis that was causing her chronic dysmenorrhea (painful menstrual periods). The operation did not disclose anything that could be helped by surgery. The extremely painful menstrual periods continued and became worse despite hormone treatments. She made thinly veiled suicidal threats, saying that when her abdominal pain was especially severe, she wanted to drive her car off the road and smash into something that would cause her to lose consciousness.

She had been married for five years, and complained that her sexual life was unsatisfactory. Little intercourse took place, and when it did the act was very painful for her. She often felt terribly depressed, was self-critical, and had overwhelming fears that some disaster would overtake her and no one would believe that she was in danger and come to her rescue. Several doctors had suggested that she might benefit from psychiatric treatment, but she rejected this advice. She insisted on a hysterectomy for the relief of pain and, before the year was out, got one.

By the time she came to my office, she was a terribly distraught young woman with a floundering marriage, abdominal pain that persisted despite a hysterectomy, frequent episodes of acute depression, and periods of claustrophobia that occurred when she was in the kitchen.

I investigated the subject of food allergy and food addiction in detail, and carefully reviewed the question of possible allergy to chemicals in the environment. I learned that she reacted to freshly manufactured plastics and rubber articles, disinfectants, air fresheners, hair sprays, paints, furniture oils, fumes from gas stoves, automobile exhausts, chlordane insecticide, and a number of foods. When she cleaned up her home environment by removing all offending household products, had her gas stove removed and the the inlet pipe that supplied her house sealed off at the meter so that no gas entered her home, and went on a rotary diet that eliminated all of the food to which she had reacted with her familiar symptoms on testing, her symptoms began to subside and in less than a month all of her complaints cleared up. The low abdominal pains that she and her doctors formerly thought were located in her uterus were actually due to allergic spasms of her lower bowel. I presented her case history in November 1967 to the International Congress of Allergology meeting in Montreal.

CASE STUDY: NAUSEA/DIZZINESS/HEADACHE/MENTAL CONFUSION

Nancy was a pretty ten-year-old girl who already was under treatment for asthma and hay fever and was known to be highly allergic to stinging insects when we met eleven years ago. Within the first ten minutes as I interviewed her with her mother, I was certain that she was allergic to environmental chemicals because she told me that she would become ill in school every time freshly printed papers were passed out in her class. She recalled that the papers usually had a strong ink odor, and most of the time the ditto fluid was not dry when she received it. She became nauseous and dizzy immediately and within a few minutes had a moderately severe headache and was unable to concentrate on her lesson. She often had these symptoms, she said, when she was in the main office when the duplicator was in operation.

I obtained the above information because I was looking for data of this nature—it was not volunteered by Nancy or her mother. It is indispensable information that would have been totally lost if I had not deliberately sought evidence regarding possible reactions to environmental exposures.

When I tested her for the presence of chemical susceptibility, I was really seeking to confirm what already was apparent from her history. The test material that I used was synthetic ethanol, which was prepared from petroleum. As in all tests, the identity of the test solution was not known to the patient, and no suggestions were made regarding any reaction to the test that I might be expecting.

Within a few minutes after the test, she became tired, was

unable to concentrate, and experienced severe visual blurring. A few minutes later she developed nausea, chills, a sensation of intense dryness in her throat, and she was unable to stand without support. She said that she was very thirsty, felt as if she were on a cloud and everything around her was much too bright to look at. I handed her a glass of cool water to relieve the dryness in her throat, and after taking a few sips she complained that I had given her "hot cola." She became very angry with me for being so mean to her. In simple terms her nervous system was confused and her perceptions were no longer correctly interpreted. She enthusiastically performed somersaults and believed she was going backward when she was going forward and vice-versa. During this period of increased activity, she struck her elbow against a wall and complained that she had hurt her knee.

Her mother was sitting next to her wearing a white blouse and a green sweater, but Nancy said that the man sitting next to her was her teacher and named a male teacher whose class she had been in two years previously; she said that he was wearing an orange jacket and a blue shirt. She placed my stethoscope in her ears and became very irritated that she could not hear any music; she threw it on the floor, saying it was broken. She did not know what day it was, and she did not recognize me, although she had been to the office many times for treatments. She said that my face looked funny and that it was yellow with purple spots moving across it. She said that she felt very cold, then became angry with a lighting fixture on the wall because the heat didn't come on while she was vigorously shaking the fixture.

As the reaction to ethanol progressed, she became restless, overenthusiastic about minor occurrences, and then showed considerable irritability. She was unable to read and, after looking at the window, stated that it was raining very hard; the day was bright and sunny. She picked up the telephone and dialed a sequence of numbers. Her mother, who was sitting next to her, heard a voice answer the phone and she took it from Nancy in order to apologize or explain to the victim what she thought was a random selection of numbers. Much to her surprise, Nancy had dialed a familiar number, and I heard her mother say, "Hello, Mother. Nancy just called you." Despite Nancy's confusion and the statement that she was playing with the radio, she had indeed dialed her grandmother but was not aware of the fact that she had done so. She took a paper towel, tore off a small piece, said that it was a piece of lettuce and that it was delicious, and began chewing it. She then tore off another piece and indicated that she was now eating a hot dog. When she appeared to have had enough, she placed the rest of the paper in a wastebasket, indicating that this was the refrigerator. A few minutes later she went back to the "refrigerator" and began to eat the paper from the wastebasket. She went over to my desk, took a piece of paper from the drawer, tore off a small part, and chewed it with wild enthusiasm. She was given a comic book to read and she pretended to do so, making a series of silly remarks that had nothing to do with the content of the story she pretended to be reading.

I discussed the significance of this prolonged reaction with her mother and made her aware of the fact that many petro-leum chemical products caused her daughter to be ill and inter-fered with many of the functions of her nervous system. Mrs. S. told me that this completely explained a peculiar incident that had occurred a few days previously. Nancy had been stand-ing on a street corner waiting to cross the road, and while waiting, she was standing next to a car with a running motor. She suddenly became confused and walked directly into the side of the car. Her mother then went on to tell me that Nancy often became quite dizzy when leaving the house for school in the morning and several times had almost fallen down the back stairs as she left the kitchen, in which there was a gas stove in operation.

Her entire reaction to this test with ethanol is documented on tape and motion picture film, with the kind permission of her family. I had the privilege of presenting a case report, along with the tape recording and motion picture documentation, to the International Congress of Allergology in 1967.

Because of the dramatic clinical evidence I was able to obtain by testing the child, the parents agreed to cooperate com-pletely with me in my suggestions for cleaning up the home environment. They removed many of the sources of indoor chemical air pollutants. The gas appliances were replaced with electric ones, and many household cleaning and maintenance materials that were petroleum byproducts were removed. This environmental change was immediately of considerable benefit; her morning dizziness disappeared along with her fatigue, and there was a striking improvement in her school performance. In addition, there was a happy development shortly after the natural gas was eliminated from her home: Her mother's arthritis of fourteen years' duration disappeared completely, and six months later, when I had a chance to test the mother for allergy to petroleum products, I was able to bring on a typical severe attack of her arthritic pains in many joints by testing Mrs. S. with a dose of ethanol similar to the one that had brought on the prolonged and bizarre reaction in her daughter.

Your Environment and Food Testing

In order to test yourself for food allergy you are going to have either to fast for five days prior to testing or to eliminate the foods in the test for five days prior to testing. During this five-day period if you clean up your home and work environment simultaneously, you can immediately decrease a tremendous allergic burden from chemicals, dusts, danders, molds, and pollens.

The results often are dramatic. If you have been suffering from migraine headaches and they are caused by fumes escaping from your gas stove as well as from a food you are eating, the pretest fast or food-elimination period *and* turning off your stove will allow your system to clean itself out and cease reacting. If you are depressed for no apparent reason and your depression is caused by animal dander or the room deodorizer you spray periodically around the house, giving the cat away and discontinuing the use of the room deodorizer for the pretest and test periods for foods may lift your cloud of depression almost miraculously.

Then, after you have tested yourself for food allergies and established a list of foods to which you are not allergic, you can test yourself at home for chemical allergies.

At-Home Test for Allergy to Air Pollutants

CLEANSE YOUR ENVIRONMENT

1. Remove *everything* from the house that has a distinct odor. In the kitchen remove everything from under the sink— all the floor and furniture polishes, oven and window cleaners, cleansers, insecticides, *everything*. In the bathroom, remove all the hair spray, nail polish and remover, scented soaps, cosmetics, deodorants. Either remove every can or tube of paint, paint thinner, glue, or oil from the utility closet, or seal up the closet and do not open it. If you are going to do it, you might as well do it right! Pack up the drugs and bandages in the medicine cabinet. Do not take *any* medicine unless it is prescribed by your doctor and it would be dangerous to your health for you to discontinue it. Do not stop your digitalis, insulin, thyroid, etc.

2. Have the gas stove turned off (at the meter if possible). Park the car outside the garage if the garage is part of the house. Turn off the gas heat. Do not use the gas dryer.

3. If you are not fasting, eat only food from a health food store if you possibly can do so. There are many chemicals in commercial supermarket food. If you cannot get to a health food store, buy only foods not wrapped in heat-sealed plastic— petroleum byproducts are trapped in the food as a result of heating the plastic to seal the package. The only packaged foods that I know about that are relatively free from pollutants in the supermarket are dry powdered skim milk, okra, frozen cooked squash, and frozen lima beans. Melon and Jerusalem artichokes are also relatively free from chemicals. Fresh fish from a small, local market is fine. Bananas, as long as they do not have large brown blazes (which means they have been chemically ripened), are fine, too.

4. Brush your teeth with sea salt or baking soda and spring water. Shave with an electric shaver. Use ice water afterwards as an astringent. Wash your hair and body in Johnson's Baby Shampoo. Take sponge baths in spring water if your tap water

is chlorinated. Use an old sheet as a shower curtain, and remove the plastic curtain and liner.

5. Cigarettes must go. Now is as good a time as any to quit. The chemicals in tobacco and in the paper the tobacco is wrapped in are lethal offenders that could seriously affect you and interfere with this entire program.

6. Wear old clothing that has been washed in Ivory soap or Rokeach kosher soap or Arm and Hammer washing soda. The test to determine which clothing is suitable for wear during this test is simple: Observe what happens when you drop a few drops of water on a garment. If the water sinks in, it is okay to wear; if it does not, put it back in a closet you will be sealing off.

7. Remove any plastic cover on the bed. If the mattress itself is plastic, cover it with layers of a blanket laundered in one of the above-mentioned soaps. Do not use a rubber or plastic foam rubber pillow. Fold a cotton sheet, blanket or towel for a pillow. Do not use polyester sheets or put towels or cotton blankets inside polyester pillowcases. Do not use an electric blanket; the wires are insulated in plastic and will emit a vapor when the blanket is heated. Seal off the closets containing clothes you should not wear.

8. Have relatives or neighbors care for your pets in their home.

9. Have a friend board all your potted plants; molds are everywhere in the soil.

10. Do not cook in aluminum pots. For some reason as yet unknown, these can cause problems in some people. Use Pyrex, Corningware, stainless steel, or cast iron pots instead. Do not burn the foods as this may result in the formation of tars. Do not fry because smoke can be a problem. Cook very slowly or cook with water. Wash dishes and pots with tap water and Ivory soap. In most cases rinsing with spring water is not necessary. Do not dry with paper towels; they are treated with chlorine bleaches. Do not use anything plastic, plates and cups included.

11. You will drink only spring water or pure well water from glass bottles during this time period. By avoiding the plastic containers that most spring water comes in, you can avoid the active chemical substances that are usually given off by the plastic itself.

Test for Chemical Susceptibility

Test one chemical when you first get up in the morning, another in midafternoon, and a third in the early evening.

Day #1 *Chlorine*

Drink 3 glasses of tap water from your kitchen or bathroom sink (your usual source).

Furniture polish

Spray your furniture polish on a rag until it is soaked. Sit 2 feet away in a small room for 15–20 minutes with the door shut.

Ammonia

Mix 1 tbs in 1 cup of water. Soak a blotter, and sit 2 feet away in a small room for 15–20 minutes.

Day #2 *Clorox*

Mix 1 tbs in 1 cup of water. Soak a blotter and sit 2 feet away in a small room for 15–20 minutes with the door shut.

Cigar

Light 3 cigars (do not smoke them) and put in an ashtray. Sit 2 feet away in a small room for 15–20 minutes with the door shut.

Moth Balls

1 tsp in an empty cup. Sit 2 feet away in a small room for 15–20 minutes.

Day #3 *Detergent*

Fill the bathroom sink with a laundry detergent and spring water. Make suds. Stay in the bathroom for 15–20 minutes.

Fresh newsprint

Buy a freshly printed newspaper and read it for 15–20 minutes. Hold it close to you

Gasoline exhaust

Sit in your driveway 10 feet behind your car with the motor running.

Day #4 *Cigarette*

Light 3 cigarettes (do not smoke them) and put in an ashtray. Sit 2 feet away in a small room for 15–20 minutes with the door shut.

Hair spray

Spray hair spray for 15 seconds in a small room. Stay there for 15–20 minutes with the door shut.

Foam rubber

Lie down for 15–20 minutes with your head on a new foam pillow or plastic foam pillow (use the kind you usually sleep on).

Day #5 *Fumes from gas stove*

Turn on the oven, close or seal off the kitchen door, and sit in the kitchen for 15–20 minutes.

Turpentine

Soak a blotter, and sit 2 feet away in a small room for 15–20 minutes with the door shut.

Perfume/cologne

Take your favorite perfume or cologne and place a few drops just under your nose for 15–20 minutes.

198

12. Try and take a week off from work if you can, or wait until vacation time to test yourself. Spending eight hours a day in an office environment filled with chemical pollutants could negate some of the benefit of being in a totally controlled home environment.

IF YOU HAVE A SEVERE REACTION

Don't forget the alkaline salts remedy (see Appendix) if your reaction is so severe you don't want to let it runs its course. Mix 2 heaping tablespoons of baking soda (sodium bicarbonate) with 1 heaping tablespoon of potassium bicarbonate, and add a heaping teaspoon of this mixture to 16 ounces of spring water. Aspirin-free Alka Seltzer Gold is also helpful and has a more pleasant taste. Take two successive doses of 1 tablet to a glass of water in place of the alkaline salts. Milk of magnesia (unflavored) may be taken (2 to 4 tablespoons) for additional relief.

WARNING: Again, if you have kidney disease or heart disease, remember that these alkaline salts contain sodium and are not to be taken unless your physician permits you to do so.

AFTER THE TEST

If you reacted to any or all of the at-home tests, you will have to make some overall changes and adjustments in your home environment to eliminate or minimize your exposure to the chemical substances that you cannot tolerate. Some of the measures are relatively easy—you can remove the foam rubber pillows from the beds, put an exhaust fan in a bathroom so you do not have to use air fresheners, clean the floors with soap and water and do not wax or polish with petroleum products.

In some situations it is impossible for a chemically susceptible person to become well until some rather expensive steps have been taken. If a family member is terribly ill from the fumes generated by the gas heating system in your home or the gas stove and laundry dryer, the most effective measure is to change to electric heat and replace the stove and dryer with electric appliances. This kind of change may cost $2,000 to $4,000 but if you weigh the cost of an unhappy and unproductive life, a broken family, walking around in a state of mental confusion, suffering from chronic discomfort such as headache with arthritis pains, or spending from $800 to $2,000 a week in a mental hospital, the importance of money is diminished. I do not advise your moving from a home that you are otherwise satisfied with. The costs of buying, selling, and moving are usually far greater than the costs of making the necessary changes in your present home.

In addition (although it is not always possible to the degree required), the work environment and the school environment should also be corrected. If you have your own office space or cubicle, you can make it a little protected oasis by prohibiting smoking, seeing that felt-tipped pens are not used (petroleum product), furniture polish is not used (more petroleum products), plants are removed (molds), the floor is not waxed, and no air freshener is employed. Copying machines should not be located in this area, several "thank you for not smoking" signs can be placed in strategic locations, and you can make certain there are no ashtrays in the room. (Last year, I was invited to the governor's office in California to discuss the role of allergy and nutritional factors in physical and mental illness. There were several "no smoking" signs in the office, but there also was an ashtray covered with a piece of cloth on a floor stand next to Governor Brown's desk. The cloth was like the birdcage covers that are used to cover pet birds for the night, and I inquired about the presence of both of the signs and the ashtray. I was told that this ashtray would be uncovered only if the President of the United States visited and required its use—no other visitors were permitted to pollute the air in the governor's office since he and several of his staff members found that tobacco smoke fumes had an adverse effect on them.)

You will be pleasantly surprised how understanding and cooperative people will be if you nicely and gently explain your problem and ask for their help with respect to the use of perfume, cologne, hair spray, etc.

Is the Water in Your Home Making You Ill?

The water? Yes, it is very possible. Most families, especially those living in cities, rely on chemically treated water supplies. I have found that there are elements in the water supplies that cause a great deal of difficulty—chlorine in particular. I am not saying that the use of chlorine is bad for a water supply. Without chlorine treatment, we would have serious trouble with important forms of waterborne disease, but there are people who are sensitive to the effects of chlorine. We add chlorine to water because it is a toxic substance able to destroy dangerous living organisms, such as the typhoid germ, which could cause disastrous epidemics. But chlorine has been known to cause many problems in chlorine-sensitive people.

SYMPTOMS FROM CHLORINATED WATER

One of my patients was a schizophrenic girl who experienced a multiplicity of symptoms when I gave her tests to determine a possible nervous system sensitivity to chlorine. She began to hyperventilate, panicked, and became depressed. After I discovered this cause-and-effect relationship between chlorine and her schizophrenia, she was ordered to avoid anything containing chlorine—city water, chlorine-containing scouring powders, chlorine laundry bleach, and chlorinated swimming pools. And, as in most cases of bio-ecologic physical and mental illness, multiple environmental factors were involved. Chlorine was one of the important causes of her illness.

In another case, a woman found her severe arthritis was linked directly to the tap water in her house; I had her fast for five days, then tested her with a drop of chlorine test solution under the tongue, and within five minutes her arthritis flared up. Another patient, a five-year-old girl who had extreme irritability combined with chronic itching, was fasted in the hospital on spring water, then tested with the chlorinated city water, and she reacted with the symptoms described above. She particularly scratched behind her knees and in front of her elbows—areas where she had had eczema for several years. She was tested with both spring water and city water, but she was never told which of these forms of water she was drinking. Shortly after taking the chlorinated tap water, she said "this is the bad water" and began to scratch frantically. She had no reaction to the spring water. At this point her mother recalled that during the previous summer, when they had been using well water exclusively, there had been no itching or scratching.

STEPS TO TAKE IF WATER IS A PROBLEM

Sensitivities to the chemicals in your drinking water are much easier to handle than you might suspect. Chlorine is usually the main offender, and this can be controlled by fairly simple measures.

You can begin by eliminating tap water in your home from the municipal water supply and substituting well water or spring water in glass bottles for drinking and cooking. In this way you can avoid many reactive substances, including chlorine and the potentially dangerous compounds that are formed when chlorine combines with organic material present in water.

A few additional steps you can take include eliminating chlorine-containing scouring powders and detergents and the use of chlorine bleach in laundering. A few crystals of sodium thiosulfate, easily obtainable at your pharmacy, may be added to your bathwater, and the chlorine will be changed to a harmless, nonodorous substance. (Do not drink the sodium thiosulfate treated water or cook in it—this is strictly for bathtub use.)

An alternative to buying spring water is to pour the chlorinated tap water into wide-mouthed bowls and expose the surface of the water to air for three days. It is not necessary to cover the water unless there is a great deal of dust or mold in the air of your home. Another option is to boil tap water for ten minutes; this removes the chlorine.

Is Mold in Your Home Making You Ill?

As if the chemicals throughout the home were not enough, there are other problem areas—house dust and molds. Whenever you have sat in a chair by a sunny window, you have probably noticed the enormous numbers of particles drifting, swirling, and dancing around in the rays of sunlight streaming through the window. These harmless-looking particles can be as insidious allergic offenders as the chemicals in the air. What you see in this golden sunlight are particles of cotton, dust, wool, linen, silk, synthetic fabrics, fragments of decaying insect bodies, and the ever present molds, of which there are thousands of species known to man.

Molds are present in the atmosphere throughout the year in varying concentrations. In fact, the only time when there is not very much mold in the air is when there has been a layer of snow (on top of the mold) covering the ground for a period of five days or longer. Molds are an important part of the never ending cycle by which organic material is broken down to simple substances that are returned to the soil to be used again. It is by the action of molds that the leaves and grass clippings in the compost pile are broken down to make fertilizer.

Molds are light; they are borne effortlessly by local winds and air currents. A twenty-mile-per-hour wind will carry them two-hundred miles in ten hours. It has been stated that the southerly wind passing over the Georgia swamps can bring molds to the middle Atlantic and New England states if the wind blows long enough. All they need to proliferate is a little moisture and darkness: a nice damp basement, some damp dust rags, perspiration-soaked shoes, grouting on the bathroom wall, a drip pan in the refrigerator, a flower pot with damp soil, a house in a wooded area that lacks sunlight and remains constantly damp, and most particularly, a house with a basement floor made of dirt or a crawl space with dirt floors so that simple capillary action can take place through the ground and draw water into the dirt areas of the house where it is dark and warm, and where the ideal environment is provided for molds to grow.

Case Study: Stuffy Nose/Itchy, Sore Palate/Difficulty Breathing

I well remember an extremely unhappy series of incidents that occurred when I was a medical student "keeping company" with a very nice young woman whose home I would often visit on weekends. Her family lived in a lovely old house situated on a piece of property that had once been a large dairy, poultry, and vegetable farm. Every time I spent a night in the upstairs bedroom that was kindly turned over to me, I became miserably uncomfortable in less than one hour. I would develop a runny, stuffy, itchy nose; the roof of my mouth would itch intensely and then become sore; my ears would become blocked; and I would spend most of the night propped up on the pillow with my mouth open because it was impossible to breathe through my nose.

Finally, I became so uncomfortable that, although I couldn't figure out what was wrong at the time, I asked if I could sleep downstairs on a sofa. All I knew was that I had to get out of that room.

Several years later, by sheer accident I solved the mystery of my nighttime miseries in the upstairs bedroom. I was looking for something in the closet of this bedroom when to my great surprise I came upon a tiny, narrow set of stairs in the far corner deep inside this dark closet. The stairs led to an attic. When I pushed back the attic trap door and took a look, I was shocked to see great piles of old, old cornstalks covered with massive quantities of molds.

Obviously, the original farmer had stored corn in the attic to feed to the cattle in the winter. I was getting a tremendous exposure to mold by sleeping in the bedroom just under the attic. The mold was constantly growing in the darkness of the attic, and spores filled the air in my bedroom. No wonder I had to get out of there, even though I couldn't initially understand why!

CASE STUDY: ASTHMA

A middle-aged woman came to me with a long history of severe asthma. I found out that she was a geranium fancier and that she had at least twenty-five potted specimens in her living room, dining room, and bedroom. I asked her to bring one of her plants to the office so that I could test the soil for molds. When she arrived for her next appointment with a very large and attractive flower pot, I could *see* the soil was covered with molds. (Since molds are microscopic, it takes a very heavy growth of molds to make them visible to the naked eye.)

I took a pinch of soil from the geranium pot, rubbed it between my fingertips from a height of about one foot over a special mold culture dish, and just let the fine dust from the pot settle on the mold-growing medium before I covered and incubated the culture. Within a matter of three to four days, the medium in the petri dish had a luxuriant growth of molds in it that would have taken at least a week or two to grow if the soil had not been so laden with molds in the first place.

I took the culture to the bacteriology laboratory of the New York Medical College, where a mycologist who specializes in growing and identifying molds studied the plate prepared from the geranium-bearing soil. He stated that there were at least eight different species of molds growing in the culture, and that he would have to perform some special tests to identify all of them, but he was positive about three of them. One of these was penicillium.

When I performed an inhalation test on this patient for bronchial sensitivity to penicillium, she had a moderately severe attack of asthma. I told her she had to make one of four choices: She could get rid of her plants; she could try repotting them in sterile soil, which would reduce her exposure to the mold for a while; she could begin a program of chemical sterilization on the soil to kill the molds, but I suspected she might also have a sensitivity to the chemicals; or I could begin a mold desensitization program on her, but I did not believe that treatments would give her the degree of protection she required because of the massive exposure to airborne molds she was constantly experiencing in her home many hours a day. In other words, I believed that the plants had to be removed from the house.

This lady immediately became disenchanted with me when I outlined these alternatives. Instead of being thrilled that one of the major causes of her serious, life-threatening asthma had been positively identified, she stormed out of my office never to return because she would not consider getting rid of her beautiful and beloved plants or participating in any repotting or chemical treatment program that could possibly affect them negatively.

A few years later, I learned from the physician who had referred her to me that she had become so sick with asthma that she ended up in the pulmonary intensive care unit of a hospital and nearly died. Before her return home from the hospital she had every last one of the plants removed from her home and had the house cleaned and aired out thoroughly.

CASE STUDY: EYE, NOSE, AND THROAT HAY FEVER SYMPTOMS

Janet S., a young housewife, came to me with typical eye, nose, and throat hay fever symptoms and told me that she was very uncomfortable out on her lawn. I tested her by having her inhale a large variety of local grass pollens; they did not cause any symptoms at all, even though my final doses were very large. I was puzzled by this completely negative reaction to the series of sniff tests for grass pollen allergy, so I reviewed the problem with her. During our second consultation I learned that she would have difficulty out on the front lawn when she raked it anywhere from two to four to five days after the lawn had been cut by her husband or one of her sons. This immediately suggested the possibility of mold allergy, and she had a series of very convincing reactions when I tested her with small quantities of powdered molds.

Upon further questioning, I learned that she was fairly uncomfortable in several places in the house and very uncomfortable in both the kitchen and the basement. Together we made a room-by-room search to determine which areas or carpets or pieces of furniture might be involved in this problem. There were two overstuffed chairs that had a mild moldy odor, but when I had her place her nose close to them and inhale as I struck the pillows, she had only mild symptoms. I thought I had the mystery of the kitchen solved when she told me that standing in front of the sink was just about the worst thing she could do. This inspired the detective in me, and with a flourish I opened the cabinet door under the sink, fully expecting to find an orange or a potato wedged in the pipes and covered with mold. To my great surprise this area was spotlessly clean, and there were no mold-bearing objects visible. So for the moment the kitchen was a mystery to me, but I refused to entertain the thought that she hated housework and had emotional reactions in her kitchen that triggered typical allergic symptoms.

Next we explored the basement, since she informed me that she was usually very uncomfortable by her washing machine. When I examined this household appliance, I found an old shoe wedged under one corner of it, and she explained that this was used to level the machine because the paving on the floor was uneven. I removed the shoe, which was covered with a thick layer of greenish-gray mildew that I scraped off and placed on a piece of paper. I held the paper underneath her nose and tapped it briskly from below while she inhaled. Within a few seconds all of her symptoms flared up, and within a few minutes her nose was completely obstructed, her eyes were red and running, and she was sneezing.

I looked about the basement for other evidence and found that there were ice skates and ski boots also covered with mold. I told her that these should be wiped off and then placed in a plastic bag and stored out in the garage. When she realized what mold looked like, she said, "I think I know what's wrong with my kitchen." We went upstairs and she lowered a matchstick bamboo curtain which had been hidden behind a decorative piece of lumber over the sink; it was immediately obvious what the problem in the kitchen was. The white cord that was part of the curtain's mechanism was covered with black and brown mold spots, and the matchsticks themselves were also covered with mold. I carefully removed this curtain from its supporting hardware, slowly rolled it up so as not to disturb the molds, and brought it out to the back-yard where once again I had Janet perform another sniff test, and she excitedly exclaimed: "That's it. That's the smell that's bothered me in the kitchen for I don't know how long." This cleared up the allergic mystery in the S. household, and I was later informed that a ceremonial bonfire had been conducted in the backyard starring the matchstick bamboo curtain. End of mystery.

STEPS TO TAKE IF MOLD IS A PROBLEM

One day a friend and I were talking about his sailboat. He said, "You know, whenever I go sailing, I develop a terrible cough which is much worse when I'm down in the cabin."

We went to his boat so I could inspect it, and the moment I stepped inside the cabin I was overwhelmed by the musty odor characteristic of mildew (molds). There was little doubt in my mind that this heavy exposure to molds was responsible for allergic irritation of his upper respiratory tract which led to his episodes of coughing. The problem was how to remove the molds for a reasonable period of time without causing a persist-ent chemical problem in the boat that might result from the use of mold-killing agents.

I remembered that a colleague of mine, the late Dr. Nathan Schaeffer, who was an expert on mold allergy, had mentioned that formaldehyde was a highly effective mold killer which gave off penetrating fumes that could be easily aired out of an area after they had done their work. So my friend and I poured an inch of formaldehyde into each of two empty coffee cans. We placed one can forward and the other can aft, and closed up the cabin tightly to seal the formaldehyde vapors inside the boat. When he returned to his boat three days later, he opened the hatchway and left the boat for about a half hour. When he returned, he took a deep breath of fresh air, entered the cabin, opened all the portholes, and left his boat until all of the residual formaldehyde fumes had aired out. Dr. Schaeffer's process was highly successful, and the boat was completely free of mold; the beneficial effect of the formaldehyde disinfection lasted for approximately two months.

This form of treatment is easily applied to single rooms, basements, and entire homes. It is only necessary that the members of the household be able to remain away from home for a long weekend and arrange to have the house well aired before the it is occupied again. Formaldehyde can be quite irritating and it is necessary to take a few simple precautions to protect the eyes and respiratory tracts of everyone in the family, not just of those individuals who might become ill due to a specific susceptibility to this substance.

The average size basement requires from four to six coffee containers or soup plates or pie pans with an inch of formaldehyde in the bottom of each. Use one container for each 12' × 15' area with a 7'–8' ceiling. If you wish to eliminate the mold in an entire house at one time, place the formaldehyde solution throughout the home, including the basement and attic, close all the windows, and stay away for two full days. Air the house out thoroughly when you return or have this done for you and do not reenter your home until there is no detectable odor of formaldehyde.* This material may be purchased at most drug stores in pint bottles. If your druggist does not keep formaldehyde in stock, he can easily obtain it for you. You will require two pint bottles of formaldehyde for every five containers that are employed in this mold disinfection procedure.

House plants should not be bothered by the fumigation process. A number of my patients have carried out this procedure and have not yet reported the loss of any plants. An additional measure for reducing the mold content of the home is to repot plants in larger containers using fresh, sterile soil—this provides a layer of mold-free soil around the entire ball of earth that surrounds the root system and stem of your plant.

By eliminating the majority of those things to which you

---

*The airing-out process can be hastened by using electric fans and by swinging several doors back and forth on their hinges, being careful not to be exposed to the fumes.

are allergic, you will *reduce your total load of allergic stresses,* and you should begin to feel much better. In fact, by freeing yourself from exposures to things to which you are allergic in your home, you may find you develop a tolerance for them when you are outside the home. It is not unusual for a food-allergic patient to be able to tolerate some or many of his food offenders when the chemical load is decreased. One of my cigarette-smoking patients reported that she was able to eat about half of the foods that made her ill within a few days after she stopped smoking.

7
Nutritional Supplements

I read about a mining engineer who became lost on an expedition in the backwoods of northern Canada and wandered for weeks trying to find his way back to civilization. Suddenly he began to have such excruciating pains in his eyes that he felt that the pain would actually drive him out of his mind. Luckily, an Indian came by and realized the engineer's plight. Although they could not understand each other's language, the Indian immediately recognized the nature of the pain this engineer was suffering from. The Indian built a small dam in a nearby stream and caught a fish and by sign language he instructed the engineer to eat the eyes of the fish. Slowly, the pain subsided and disappeared completely. Later, the engineer learned that fish eyes are one of the richest sources of vitamin A known to man. A "primitive" Indian whose knowledge was based on tribal lore provided the kind of information that was necessary to control this excruciatingly painful vitamin deficiency disease of the eye.

The Indians in Peru used to raise guinea pigs because the guinea pig, living on greens, was able to synthesize tremendous amounts of vitamin C. Also, some natives of South America would make trips from the mountains down to the seashore to gather seaweed, which was rich in minerals. The tribesmen did not know exactly why guinea pigs or seaweed were good for them, but some ancestors had made these discoveries about nutrition and the information was passed down through the ages. The end result was that the tribes got adequate amounts of vitamin C and minerals that were lacking in their inland diets. In some primitive societies before a young woman and her future husband got married, they were put on a special diet in anticipation of bearing children.

In recent civilization, as a means of having a ready supply of food, vegetables were cultivated and domesticated animals were grazed on the same land for many years. Surrounding the farmer's fields were acres of uncut trees, and dividing the fields were long stretches of hedgerows in which birds nested and raised their young. These birds lived on the insects and pests that were in the vicinity and in this manner the natural symbiotic balance was maintained. The soil was kept rich; crops grew; the cows, chickens, and horses had grain; and the farmer and his family had food. Every season the process began anew until the land was no longer productive. At that point one of three things happened: Entire families packed up their belongings and moved to other areas, or they plowed under the crops and used the time-honored method of allowing the land to lie fallow until it replenished itself, or they rotated their crops.

A major problem developed in the mid-nineteenth century when a German agricultural chemist named Liebig got the idea that everything required by a plant could be found in the mineral ash of that plant. It was because of his influence that synthetic fertilizers with a nitrogen, potassium, and phosphorus (NKP) content became widely used.* The synthetic fertilizers, however, were incomplete. They could cause rapid and uniform growth of a crop, but they could not provide all the nutrients a healthy crop required.

Another major problem began with the Industrial Revolution in this country. A machine could clear more land than a farmer, his family, and any helpers could clear in ten times as much time. Huge machines rolled across the land, plowing and fertilizing. The amount of land devoted to crops increased; the forests and hedgerows began to disappear. *The birds left;* they no longer had as many places to nest. *The insects and pests stayed;* they multiplied without the birds to keep them in reduced numbers. And therefore insecticides and pesticides began to be used across the fields. These chemicals left toxic residues in the

*Balfour, E. B. *The Living Soil* (New York: Devlin, 1948).

food that were totally foreign to our body chemistry. Not only did we eat the food, but we fed our animals with it and then ate them. We took the seeds from this contaminated food and planted them for the following year's crop.

Meanwhile, along with the insects and pests, the soil began to lose its microbial life—those tiny, very much alive organisms with which the rootlets of a plant interact to get a major part of their nutrition. Lacking these microbes to draw on, the plants' nutritional value decreased. Inferior seeds from nutritionally inferior plants were sowed now in inferior soil. Perpetuating a vicious cycle, we again ate the plants, and fed our animals on them, and then ate the animals.

Adding to this problem, canning, drying, freezing, smoking, and pasteurization took their toll on the vitamin and mineral content of food. With antifungal drugs, antioxidants, anticaking and foaming agents, blenders, bleaches, and antibacterial agents used to prolong the edibility of plants and meat added, man was truly under an "assault"—and he no longer has the necessary nutrients at his disposal to be healthy enough to counter this attack on a simple biochemical level.

It is impossible to eliminate this chemical pollution of our food supply. Washing the outside of a vegetable or fruit is almost a worthless gesture. When a crop has been sprayed eight, ten, twelve, or fifteen times from the blossom stage until there is fully developed ripe fruit, you cannot get rid of the spray by washing, scraping, or peeling—the insect and mold-killing agents are also in the pulp. They have permeated the food as it has been growing.

While all this trouble with crops was happening, we also developed the problem of agricultural "runoff." The insecticides and herbicides (weed killers) and synthetic fertilizers, getting washed into our streams and lakes, may very well end up in the reservoirs that supply our drinking water. Now, not only are we eating food contaminated with insect and weed poison, we are also drinking water that has been chemically polluted with these toxic agents. Throwing in some industrial wastes spewing out of smokestacks all over the country as well as being discharged into our streams, and we are not only eating and drinking pollutants, we are also breathing them.

We are virtually defenseless. For several generations we have lacked nutritious food. As a result, we have begun to deteriorate on a biochemical level, and have undergone important chemical changes in our bodies. We get headaches or become depressed for "no apparent reason"; we get heart palpitations seemingly "out of the blue"; we get weak and fatigued, and yet we have had sufficient sleep; we get asthma and "no one can find the cause." All of these complaints and many more can result from a series of chemical imbalances in a pollution-exposed body suffering from a lack of the vitamins and minerals it needs in order to remain healthy.

Now and then we hear "a voice crying in the wilderness" about the benefits of vitamins and minerals and good nutrition and proper preparation of foods. Adele Davis, the nutritionist, was often maligned by physicians but she was on the right track. So are those men and women who properly employ megavitamin therapy. All have part of the solution to mankind's health problems.

But just eating the "right" foods that are currently available will not do it. The "right" foods no longer have the essential substances that our bodies need to function. A so-called properly balanced diet may look attractive on the plate, but it leaves the body hungry for what it needs most of all to sustain itself—the vitamins and minerals that are not present in the foods, which, in addition, contain toxic residues that interfere with important body processes. Over half the calories consumed by people in the United States, Great Britain, and other industrialized nations have large quantities of empty carbohydrate calories, a fact that probably explains the prevalence of degenerative diseases. There is a striking contrast in the health of white mice fed on enriched white bread and the health of mice raised on bread baked from freshly ground whole wheat.

Nature demands that what is taken out of the soil must be returned to it. Human health can't be any better than the quality of the food eaten. It is as simple as that. If the food has been chemically treated and processed, the quality of the food is changed. If the fruit and vegetables were grown in poor soil, the food has got to be deficient in vitamins, minerals, and trace elements.

Seeing an illness in a different perspective is a real problem in the medical community. There seems to be a mental block against taking what is accepted as an established disorder and considering that it might also represent a working model of other similar disorders. Thinking along these lines is referred to as "inductive reasoning," in which a specific observation leads an individual to develop a general concept or concepts.

Pellagra, a vitamin B_3 deficiency disease, provides us with a classic example of, to put it gently and kindly, constricted thinking on the part of many physicians. Medical students know pellagra as the Disease of the 4Ds. They are dermatitis, diarrhea, dementia (another word for psychotic behavior), and death. My bio-ecologically-oriented psychiatric colleague, Dr. William Philpott, former research director of the Fuller Memorial Sanitarium in South Attleboro, Massachusetts, who is presently located in Spencer, Oklahoma, reviewed all of the serious mental symptoms that had been described in proven cases of pellagra. He found that *every form* of psychotic behavior that was reported in the psychiatry literature had been seen in pellagra.

Once it was discovered why people had pellagra, it was possible to effect a complete cure of their psychotic behavior with appropriate use of vitamin B_3, and good health was restored by appropriate additional nutritional measures. As the result of a vitamin deficiency, these individuals had a serious but simple-to-treat disease of the nervous system profoundly affecting their mental state. After this initial discovery was reported in 1939, another group of researchers studied patients who did not have pellagra but had psychotic disorders, and much to their surprise they found that many of these patients were also improved with vitamin B_3 therapy—that was almost forty years ago. (Don't be surprised. Remember, penicillin sat on the shelf "undiscovered" for almost twenty years while millions of people died because no one thought to question why no bacteria were growing near the penicillium molds on culture plates in the laboratory!)

To most physicians, the fact that a nutritional deficiency such as pellagra causes psychotic behavior and can be cured by the administration of vitamin B_3, and that "psychoses" can be cured by vitamin B$_3$, does not appear to be important in relation to mental illness. To me it was a revelation. *I* do not regard pellagra as an uncommon nutritional disorder rarely seen by the majority of physicians in practice. I see pellagra and the lack of vitamin B$_3$ as providing insight into the possible causes of many types of illness in which nutritional deficiencies may be responsible for disorders of the nervous system as well as the rest of the body. Obviously this suggests that these disorders may be cured by relatively simple nutritional means instead of being controlled temporarily by the use of potent and often dangerous drugs, or completely misunderstood and subjected to endless sessions of psychiatric talk therapy or shock treatments.

It is well known that a severe form of thiamine deficiency known as beriberi, which is associated with heart failure, an enlarged heart, and inflammation of the nerves (neuritis), dramatically responds to treatment with thiamine—vitamin B$_1$.

Is it not reasonable to suppose that some individuals in heart failure might be improved to some degree by additional thiamine if their dietary intake of vitamin B$_1$ has been marginal or below their specific individualized need for this substance? Should any individuals in heart failure be denied the slightest possible benefit that might come from the use of this widely acknowledged nontoxic and essential nutritional factor? Nothing is to be lost and a great deal might be gained, but it is a rare physician who would even consider that vitamin supplementation might be in any way effective in a case of heart failure due to both known and unknown causes.

The limeys knew that scurvy could be cured by eating limes before it was known that there were such things as vitamins. But one of the interesting things about the British sailors of long ago is that before they knew about lime eating, some sailors would get scurvy and others would not! Men would ship out and only some would come back a year or two later. Although all of them suffered from vitamin C deprivation in their diets, there were those who survived and whose unpleasant job it had been to bury at sea the sailors who died from scurvy.

When a group of people take high doses of vitamin C, some of them will "spill" large amounts of it in their urine, and others will pass little or no vitamin C after taking the same doses.

Groups of athletes—men free of illness and in top physical condition—have been tested with different vitamins in the same manner. Each man was given specific vitamins at specific dose levels, and as the dosage was increased for each man, each of the vitamins began to appear in the urine. Some of the athletes took twenty times as much of a given vitamin as the others took before it was passed in their urine. The range of dosage was enormous—up to a 2000 percent difference in their apparent needs.

From studies like this we have come to realize that we do not know what the optimal vitamin requirements are for most individuals. We do know that the dose of vitamin C that is required for maximum health in animals (so they will be vigorous and fertile and have normal offspring) seems to be one hundred times as great as the dose that is required to prevent the *appearance* of a vitamin deficiency state. What is going on within the body between the level of vitamin abundance and the appearance of a deficiency disease as the vitamin availability drops through the range of adequacy is uncertain, but it is highly probable that some of our mental and physical ailments begin to manifest themselves at levels that are suboptimal.

The Case for Synthetic Vitamins

For years the proponents of natural vitamins have been taking on the advocates of synthetic vitamins, and vice versa. Usually, the main argument against synthetic vitamins is that although laboratory-produced synthetic vitamins are chemical duplicates of the known vitamins, there may be other important vitamins or vitaminlike substances in combination with trace elements that have yet to be discovered and that may be found only in association with naturally occurring vitamins. Vitamin B_1 was discovered first and subsequently vitamin B_2, vitamin B_3, and so forth. The entire vitamin B complex has existed for hundreds of thousands of years and was consumed by our ancestors for many centuries before modern-day scientists discovered it. These essential nutrients were always there and we simply did not know that they were around. Perhaps there are others—we just don't know yet.

I agree in principle with those who believe in natural vitamins, but in practice I have found it necessary to use the chemical duplicates of these naturally occurring nondrug diet supplements. Megavitamin therapy, which is indispensable in mental illness and some other conditions, would not be possible without large amounts of economically priced synthetically manufactured replicas of these essential substances. Moderate doses of vitamins would also be far too expensive for most people if natural vitamins were employed exclusively.

Dr. Roger J. Williams, the director of research for the Clayton Foundation in Texas, is one of the world's leading biochemists and a former president of the American Chemical Society. Among his many accomplishments is the discovery and identification of the chemical structure of pantothenic acid. Pantothenic acid was isolated in his laboratory through the processing of hundreds of pounds of liver. With a great deal of time and effort, less than one teaspoon was isolated and identified at a cost of $20,000. It is clear that it is economically impossible for an average person to purchase this material derived from natural sources at a cost of perhaps $20 or more per milligram each day. It is also obvious that no one could eat the quantities of liver that would be required daily for megavitamin therapy with pantothenic acid. However, after Dr. Williams worked out the chemical structure of pantothenic acid, he was able to synthesize it in an economical manner in his laboratory. Now for a few pennies we can manufacture what formerly represented $20,000 worth of naturally derived pantothenic acid; we would not be able to have it at all if we had to rely on "natural" sources.

Also, not all "natural" vitamins are completely natural. The United States government permits the word "natural" to be used on a label if some *portion* of the product comes from a natural source. One of the most misleading labels that comes to mind is the type that reads "Rose Hips Vitamin C" or "Vitamin C from Rose Hips and other natural sources." Those "other sources" mean corn, a natural substance from which vitamin C is manufactured in enormous quantities in chemical laboratories. Also, natural vitamins may be derived from sources that have been contaminated by various toxic chemical agents such as insecticides, pesticides, and herbicides, which are employed during the raising of the food sources. Also, even though some of the natural vitamins are said to be grown in organic soil, it is practically impossible to eliminate the contaminants of organic food sources employed in the production of natural vitamins with the kind of overwhelming contamination that is present everywhere at this time. Contamination certainly can be reduced and the quality of the soil may be improved, but despite Herculean efforts to get rid of them, these stubborn chemicals persist in the soil for very long periods of time.

It all boils down to a matter of definitions. Synthetic vitamins are manufactured products that duplicate naturally occurring nutrients that the body needs. Synthetic vitamins combined with minerals that are produced in a chemical laboratory are concentrated nutrients that duplicate the chemical structure of these essential elements which was determined after they were isolated from natural sources. In one form of synthetic multiple vitamin and mineral tablets, a single tablet contains all of the known nutrients and three of them can provide you with the minimum daily requirement that has been established for some nutrients along with what is an educated guess for a minimum daily requirement of those substances for which the daily need has not yet been determined—and all very economically. That's why I prefer synthetic over "natural."

VITAMIN AND MINERAL SUPPLEMENT

In my opinion one of the best of the recent developments in the field of nutritional supplementation is Dr. Roger Williams' vitamin and mineral formula, which represents his present thinking based on all of the work he has done in nutrition. He published his formula after developing what he believed to be ideal daily maintenance doses of vitamins and minerals. The Vitamin and Mineral Insurance Formula, as it is called, contains all of the known nutrients that adults and children require to meet their minimum requirements by supplementing those nutrients present in the average civilized diet.

At the present time, there is only one laboratory that faithfully reproduces his formula. It is Bronson Pharmaceuticals,* 4526 Rinetti Lane, LaCanada, California 91011. The best way to get this excellent nutritional product is for you to order it directly from the manufacturer. The tablets are starch- and sugar-free, and they contain no artificial coloring or flavoring. They are available in bottles of 100 and 250. There is a considerable saving if the larger size is purchased. A tasty chewable tablet was recently prepared for children and older individuals who are not able to swallow pills. Dr. Williams' insurance formula will supply you with what he considers to be the average minimum daily requirements for all vitamins and mineral substances that are presently known.

EXTRA VITAMIN C

In conjunction with the vitamin and mineral insurance formula, I prescribe additional vitamin C. The minimum daily requirement of vitamin C will protect an individual against the vitamin C deficiency disease, scurvy, but much greater amounts of this wonderful substance are required for optimal health and resistance to allergies and infections. Animal studies indicate that the minimum daily dose of vitamin C in health should be 4 grams (4000 mg). Under stress, animals with the capacity to make their own vitamin C will make three to four times as much, and therefore doses of 12 to 16 grams (12,000 to 16,000 mg) have been given to thousands of patients. In very severe virus infections, patients have been successfully treated with doses of 40 to 60 grams a day by Dr. Carl Klenner of North Carolina.

One of my friends at the Johns Hopkins University Hospital told me about the use of vitamin C in the case of an eight-year-old boy who had a serious bone infection (osteomyelitis) that

*The company states that orders are processed on the day they are received and sent by United Parcel Service. Dr. Williams has no financial interest in this product. He originated and then published his formula to present his ideas on nutritional supplementation to the medical community, and it was Bronson Pharmaceuticals who decided to make it available.

resisted every antibiotic that was tried. His infection was rapidly brought under control by vitamin C in doses of 5 grams per day. When everything appeared to be normal and he was free of pain and fever, the vitamin C was discontinued. Within a few days his symptoms returned. Treatment with mother nature's super antibiotic, vitamin C, was resumed with excellent results once again, but this time the treatment period was extended and his antibiotic resistant bone infection was cured.

Studies of individual vitamin C requirements have been performed in a number of disorders. Different individuals were given various "loading doses" of this vitamin to see how much each person could take before vitamin C would begin to appear in the urine. It is believed that the body uses all of the vitamin C that it needs before any is excreted through the kidneys. It is not uncommon for 8- to 10-gram doses to be taken without recovering any vitamin C from the urine of patients given a loading test.

DESICCATED LIVER

The liver therapy I employ in my practice consists of dye-free (on my special request) capsules filled with desiccated (powdered dry) liver. It is imported from Argentina because the cattle there are grazed on grass that is not sprayed with insecticides and the livers of these animals do not have any toxic chemical residues in them. This is an important factor since the liver is the major detoxifying organ of the body and all toxic substances that are absorbed after entering the intestinal tract must pass through the liver before entering the general circulation. In addition, the liver I prescribe is not treated chemically during its preparation for human consumption. The fat is removed mechanically and not by the use of chemical solutions. This Argentina beef liver is tested by the manufacturer for the presence of any possible harmful residues.

The particular brand of desiccated liver that I recommend is dried at body temperature. The liver preparations made by other reputable manufacturers meet the same standards of purity but they are dried at a higher temperature (140°F), and I believe that there may be some important changes in the nutritional properties of the final liver product because of the exposure to heat. I want my patients to have all of the possible benefits they can obtain from liver therapy and some as yet unknown factor(s) may be affected by the heating process.

The only product I am familiar with that is similar to raw organically raised liver is prepared by the Rawl Chemical Company of West Palm Beach, Florida. It takes a modest number of capsules to do the nutritional job. My patients are instructed to take from 5 to 8 of the dye-free capsules, supplied in bottles of 500, three times a day.

The Case for Organic Food

Why do the Hunzas live to be 120 or older and remain in good health, free of cancer? Why do the Bantu have so little cancer of the bowel, if any? How is it that the Aleutian women and many other so-called primitives have easy labors with a minimum of discomfort and are able to take up their household duties the same day or the next day after delivering their babies? Why do we have diseases of civilization? Why do we have such magnificent physical specimens in people who follow their ethnic wisdom with respect to eating and living?

Originally, when mankind lived a simpler life, he ate more frequently and a great deal more bulk at each meal than he does today. He had to. Unlike civilized man, primitive man did not get the concentrated empty calories that modern man gets from sugar-saturated foods and refined starches. He had to rely on getting the calories he needed to maintain his weight by constantly foraging for roots, nuts, berries, fresh fruit and vegetables; by catching fresh fish; by hunting fresh game. The vitamins, minerals, and trace elements he needed were supplied in their natural form.

Today we have major problems with our food supply. As you walk down the produce aisles in the supermarket, you look at what appear to be healthy, fresh fruits and vegetables, but what you are seeing are vegetables and fruits that are waxed to look pretty and retain their moisture, oranges dyed to look ripe and vital. As you push your cart past the meat section, you may believe all those bright red slabs of beef are highly nutritious, but what you are seeing may be pumped full of red dye to convince you it is fresh. A quick turn to the baking goods section will place you directly in front of refined, "enriched" white flour and refined cane sugar. They may do an excellent job of becoming an attractive cake in the oven, but they certainly are deficient in vitamins and minerals.

Vitamins and minerals combine with proteins and some special sugars to form thousands of enzymes which are called nature's catalysts because they are necessary to keep the body's basic biochemical machinery in operation. The body must manufacture its enzymes from materials taken in as part of the foods in the daily diet and if vitamins and minerals—the enzyme building materials—are absent from the food, these incomplete starches and empty refined sugars rob the necessary vitamins and minerals from the body's limited supply.

Thus, refined foods are eaten at great expense to the body economy. They are merely providing a semi-nutritious kind of bulk along with some "empty" calories that fill you up, satisfy your hunger, and give you instant energy but not much in the way of materials for growth and tissue repair.

An additional word about the term "enriched." This is another form of deception practiced on the public. When whole grain wheat is processed so that its bran is removed along with its extremely important wheat germ and the resulting flour is bleached, a great deal of its food value is lost forever. The term "enriched" is applied because a few vitamins are added, but the original vitamin content and minerals are never replaced. No enriched white bread will ever come near the nutritional qualities of a bread made from whole wheat flour.

For the present, I believe that the best way to provide yourself with the "unknown" vitamins, minerals, and trace elements is to eat as close-to-naturally-grown complete foods as possible. I realize the soil is going to be contaminated with chemicals and probably lacking in minerals and some organic materials, but that is what we have to work with at this time. Until the environment is replenished and put back into balance, we have no choice! At least you have a chance of eating relatively chemical-free food with many, if not all, of the necessary vitamins, minerals, and trace elements. I know it is more expensive, and I realize the health food stores are often not as conveniently located as the local supermarket, but it is crucial that organic or at least less chemically polluted food be eaten if you and your family are to be as healthy as possible.

In December 1976 in a landmark decision reported in the *Wall Street Journal,* the United States Tax Court ruled on the tax-deductible status of organic foods prescribed by a physician. The decision was in favor of the claimants, Dr. Theron G. Randolph and Janet M. Randolph, who were permitted to deduct one-half of their total organic food bill as a medical expense.

The Case for Eating Uncooked Food

When someone, somewhere discovered fire and got the idea that he could cook vegetables, meat, or a neighbor, he began to change the course of nature's dietary plan. He has been in trouble ever since. Substances are formed from foods during the cooking that are totally alien to the human system and what it was designed to handle. Heating sugar creates foreign substance and caramelizes it, making tars. Browning meat creates tars all over the meat. Nothing like these tars exists in nature. And once proteins and carbohydrates and fats are heated, they can turn into substances that are alien to the human (or animal) body.

In terms of diet, if we think of man's primary biological apparatus, we should be thinking in terms of such foods as were available to our ancestors. Fruits and vegetables should be organically grown so that they are as nutritious and free from chemical residues as possible, and they should be eaten raw whenever possible. If they are going to be cooked, they should be steamed to help retain the natural vitamins and enzymes that are lost during more intense cooking. And the water that has been used for steaming should be saved for its mineral content and used throughout the diet for soups and gravies. Meat, poultry, and fish should not be fried. Chemically susceptible individuals should avoid exposing their food to the combustion fumes of natural gas, especially in an oven or under the gas broiler. Adele Davis and other authors involved in as-close-to-natural-as-possible diets have published many recipe books on just how to go about cooking to preserve as much of the nutritional value of foods as possible. Read them.

The more we operate in harmony with nature and accept the pattern nature established for us, the better off we will be. Frankly, it is a near miracle that we have gotten away with violating nature's laws for so long.

8
Fasting

Stop eating and fast. As harsh as that advice may sound, fasting on spring water is the quickest way to allow your body to begin to cleanse itself of all the food residues (and chemical residues in the food and water) simultaneously. And believe it or not, fasting is not difficult. Initially, because you are used to eating at certain times of the day (or all day long in some cases), you will probably experience a moderate degree of hunger, but within a day or two at the most, your body will quickly adjust to not having ingested food on which to draw and will turn to its own reserves for what it needs to keep you going.

For a person with the chronic addictive form of food allergy, symptoms may flare up on the second or third day of fasting as the body begins to undergo withdrawal effects from the foods to which one is addicted. A two-tablespoon dose of unflavored milk of magnesia or a heaping teaspoon of a combination of two parts of baking soda (sodium bicarbonate) and one part of potassium bicarbonate in a large glass (12 to 16 ounces) of spring water will relieve many of these symptoms and greatly reduce the feeling that you simply must have apple pie, a huge glass of milk, a hunk of bread, a chocolate bar, a cup of coffee, or an alcoholic drink. In fact, I have known people on a fast who found that they could for the first time give up cigarette smoking easily. Why? Because by the second or third day of the fast, their body had begun to eliminate the tobacco residue and chemicals with which it had been saturated for years. These chemicals are associated with raising, curing, and flavoring tobacco, and with the production of paper in which the cigarettes are wrapped. As the level of tobacco and chemical residues in the body decreases, it becomes easier to resist going to the store to buy another pack of cigarettes.

I am not recommending that you stop eating permanently! Far from it. It usually takes about five days for the body to do a pretty thorough job of cleansing. (I fasted six days myself, lost only five or six pounds during that time, did not feel hungry or weak, and was able to exercise daily.) Once the cleansing process is in progress, tremendous changes will begin to take place in your body. Fasting is not starving. When you stop eating, your body turns to its own food reserves. Dr. George F. Cahill of the Harvard Medical School has identified a protein-sparing mechanism that is "turned on" automatically when your body no longer can rely on an immediate supply of food. During the first day or two of fasting, your body loses protein very quickly, but then that protein-sparing switch is thrown on. It takes a long time for a healthy individual to deplete his body of its reserves enough for starvation to begin. Using its own built-in stand-by system, surpluses and nonvital supplies are used up before essential life-supporting elements are touched.

I know of people (notably those who are particularly obese) who were able to fast on juices for many months, literally living off their own reserves without any health problems. I have observed spring water fasts that ranged from five to twenty-one days. Quite simply, as long as you have water, you just do not need food to survive if you have any reserves to draw on at all. And the bottom line of those "fasting" reserves is much deeper than the average person suspects. Remember the rugby players who were lost in the Andes after a terrible plane crash on the snow-covered mountain? Panic-stricken, they thought they would starve to death from lack of food. So after much soul searching and crisis of conscience, they felt they had no alternative but to eat the victims of the plane crash if they were to survive. They really did not have to do anything of the sort. They had all the water they needed to sustain them in the form of clean, fresh snow. They had had a small food supply on board the crashed plane that they used up prior to resorting to temporary cannibalism, but eating these morsels of food only made their hunger worse. If they had completely cut themselves off from food, their constant hunger would have abated quickly. Instead, by rationing food they kept the body's emergency switches turned off, so they were constantly hungry, began to be depleted of protein, and began to starve. After all, Ralph Flores and Helen Klaben were stranded in a wilderness near the Arctic in 1963 for seven weeks without food. Their diet consisted of nothing but melted snow. When they emerged from their trial, they were in good condition and their crash injuries had healed. If they had had anything to eat during that seven-week period, they probably would have died of protein deficiency like the many Biafrans who tried to eke out an existence on the starchy roots of the cassava plant.

Once you are out of the "habit" of eating, you become aware of just how much time you spend eating and thinking about eating. Hours can be spent in a single day dawdling over coffee and breakfast, munching on a snack in the late morning, eating lunch, another snack in the late afternoon, preparing dinner, picking away at a snack in the late evening. Once you have stopped eating, you begin to realize how much eating is a social activity when you are just plain bored, how many times you ate just out of habit when you weren't even hungry, and how much you ate because you were at a restaurant or a delicious no-limit buffet and you felt you were paying for it all anyhow! As well as providing your body with an opportunity to clean itself out, fasting provides a fascinating chance to assess your eating habits —to understand the difference between what you eat routinely or addictively and the amount of food sufficient to fulfill your body's daily requirement of energy, bulk, and vitamins and minerals.

The outer portion of the adrenal gland (cortex) reacts to stress by releasing hormones. The degree of stress can be determined by measuring the amount of hormones released. Fasting does not produce any increase in adrenal cortical activity at all. It gives the entire digestive tract a complete rest from its normal continuous activity, and this system becomes almost free of the huge numbers of bacteria that are always present there. Fasting gives the entire body, including the central nervous system, a tremendous respite from having to deal with allergic responses.

It is remarkable just how much better most people begin to

feel during a fast. One by one or together, the patient's chronic
symptoms may flare and then subside until, at the end of four
to five days, for the first time in his life, he is greatly relieved
or completely free of any symptoms at all. Many of my patients
with chronic nasal and sinus conditions suddenly are free of
their postnasal drip and are able to breath freely and easily. One
patient was shocked to smell the stench of urine in a subway
underpass in New York City on the fourth day of her fast.
Although she had walked through that underpass almost every-
day twice a day during the workweek, she had never been
aware of any odors. And when she got home, for the first time
she was able to taste foods as they really taste, not as they
half-taste when sense of smell has been partially lost. Another
patient suddenly had her chronic and painful arthritis symptoms of twenty years' duration diminish in intensity (after an
initial flare-up), until by the end of seven days she could move
her always stiff fingers freely. Asthma and migraine headaches
have come and then dramatically gone; muscular pains and
chronic itching have flared, then subsided; irritability, restlessness, and depression have increased and then completely disappeared as if by magic. The pain, bloating, gas, and diarrhea of
colitis—often diagnosed as a psychosomatic condition: emotional spastic colitis—clears up; and "nervous," frequently and
urgently emptying urinary bladders are at rest. Fatigue, weakness, and mental confusion are replaced by a sense of well-being
and mental clarity. Slow, sluggish, slurred, and hard to understand jerking or stuttering speech has become normal, while
spelling errors and horrible penmanship return to normal.

Devotees of fasting who are not aware of the fact that there
are withdrawal symptoms associated with some forms of allergies call these physical and mental upheavals "a healing crisis,"
and they are right. As Dr. Alexis Carrel, the Nobel Prize winner
said, "Fasting purifies and profoundly modifies our tissues." And
it does. At the end of five or more days of fasting, a "new"
person can emerge*—one who is clear-eyed, mentally alert,

---

*Physically, many people who fast begin to change visibly at the end of the
first or second day as any allergic edema due to generalized and localized water
retention begins to be released. I have seen people lose from ten to fifteen or
more pounds on a five-day fast—far more than they could possibly have lost if

and symptom-free, with a whole new perspective on life and, for the first time, a realization of just how good he or she can feel. A chemically allergic person may take two or three weeks, possibly longer, to become free of the long-term effects of many years' accumulation of environmental chemical agents. The degree of improvement during the first week of fasting depends on the amount of an individual's accumulated food and chemical allergic loads, but just five days of fasting can make a dramatic difference.

Dramatic Allergic Reactions

The original studies by Dr. Herbert Rinkel (confirmed by my colleagues and me through testing ourselves and our patients) demonstrated that if you avoid a food to which you are allergic for a period of at least four to five days, after the fourth day you will most likely become acutely sensitive to the food you gave up if you were allergic to it in the first place. Fasting creates an excellent atmosphere for testing for food allergy. The chronic reactions are converted into diagnostically important acute reactions. This, of course, is the basis of the testing technique discussed throughout this book.

If you fast, and I know that many readers can do so without risk, you will be able to discover dramatically the types of symptoms food allergies and chemical sensitivities have been causing you. If instead you eat foods to which you are allergic right up to Day #1 of any of the diets throughout this book, you will probably have a reaction to them when you test them, but your allergic reaction may not have sufficient impact to *prove* to you the importance of chronic food allergy in your physical and mental state.

Initially, allergic individuals who are fasting may experience an increase in their usual symptoms. Most allergic people have withdrawal symptoms which make them *feel worse before they*

---

they had not been retaining a considerable amount of fluids. Ankles and hands thinned, bellies trimmed, cheeks hollowed, lips and eyelids flattened.

begin to feel better, and for that reason, it may be dangerous for people with serious disorders like bronchial asthma, epilepsy, or severe dizzy spells, as well as suicidal tendencies, to fast and to have a series of withdrawal reactions that could make their problems seem worse. In these cases, medical supervision is absolutely necessary. However, for the most part, fasting is a safe procedure that has been used for thousands of years for health and religious purposes without ill effects. For many, the health advantages of therapeutic fasting far outweigh the disadvantages of having to forgo eating for less than one week. If you want to determine exactly which factors in your diet you are allergic to, you might as well do it the most accurate way—fast.

How to Fast

You can begin a fast any time during the week, but I recommend starting on a Thursday evening by skipping dinner and drinking spring water from a glass container.* If you begin to fast on a Thursday evening, it should not be too difficult for you to get through the work day on Friday just being hungry, so long as you are not highly addicted to foods. But once the initial hunger stage passes and your body shifts gears and begins to undergo withdrawal symptoms, there may be a few days when you would much rather be in your own home and able to relax.

Take a mild laxative like milk of magnesia (unflavored) or citrate of magnesia after your last meal, and every other day during the fast. Those food and chemical residues from your diet are in your intestinal tract along with waste material, and there are only two ways you are going to get rid of them: through your kidneys when you urinate and through the lower intestines when you defecate. If you allow the waste material to remain there, your body will be drawing and replacing fluid along the intestinal tract that contains these food and chemical

---

*Spring water in plastic containers may be contaminated by petroleum by-products that get into the water from the chemically derived plastic.

residues. So help eliminate them periodically. Actually, if during the fast you find you do feel weak and listless or get any of your old symptoms, take two to four tablespoons of unflavored milk of magnesia and you may feel better very quickly.

Keep drinking spring water. The first thing you may notice is that every time you think about food, you will reach for the bottle of spring water. Some people go through a gallon or more the first day, but after that intake usually drops off. Bear in mind that you *need* to drink a large volume of spring water if you are to wash out the food and chemical residues in your body. Keep a good supply of bottled spring water on hand. Don't run out; it is often too tempting to take "just a little" tap water instead of going to the store. One glass of tap water that contains substances you are sensitive to can seriously interfere with the outcome of the fast.

Take it easy. You may experience a rapid weight loss because accumulated "allergic edema" fluid is finally released. Vigorous exercise and standing up too suddenly can leave your head spinning.

Keep warm. You may find you feel a bit chilly when everyone else is warm. It is not unusual. Just put on another sweater, or use an additional blanket on the bed.

Avoid extremes in temperature. Hot baths or showers or saunas can leave you feeling limp and weak; extreme cold can drain your body as it fights to keep warm.

Put your medications back in the medicine cabinet. Your body is trying to clean itself out and become stabilized simultaneously. Check with your physician and ask if you may omit any of your current medications for two weeks (five days of fasting plus the period of time for your particular food test schedule). Let's try to get rid of *all* the chemicals in your body if we can, and see how it fares.

Do not smoke. This is an excellent opportunity to discard a very unhealthy habit. While fasting, many patients have found it possible to give up cigarettes when no other method has worked. Why? As I mentioned earlier in the chapter, cigarette tobacco and the papers cigarettes are wrapped in are saturated in all sorts of chemicals. Since you are smoking habitually, it is likely that you have an addictive allergy to either the tobacco or the chemicals. By eliminating *all* the possible allergic factors simultaneously (the foods, beverages, chemicals, and—if you are participating in an environmental control program at the same time—the air pollutants and airborne pollens, molds, danders, and dust), you may find it is not anywhere near as difficult as you thought it would be finally to stop smoking.

Do not eat a single morsel of food or drink one sip of anything but spring water. One bite of a cookie, or a sip of diet soda will disrupt your metabolism. Instead of continuing to utilize body fat, your body may turn back to incoming food for what it needs.

Do not use toothpaste or mouthwash. Sorry. You must brush your teeth with sea salt or baking soda because toothpaste and mouthwash contain active substances that will be absorbed just like food. Bad breath can get to be a problem while you are fasting, but once your system is cleaned out, the bad breath should disappear, too. If you get a film over your tongue, brush your tongue, too. No tap water for rinsing; this is strictly a spring water fast.

Do not take vitamins or mineral supplements. Omit them for the duration of the fast and during the food and chemical tests. Taking anything other than water into your stomach might trigger hunger and confuse your body again about which direction it should be going in to get its energy.

Take handwriting samples. Do it at nine in the morning, at noon, three o'clock, six, and finally at about ten in the evening every day to see if there are any changes. Often there are. I had one patient who noticed a dramatic change in the penmanship in her checkbook and on her checks over the course of a fast. By the fifth day, her notoriously illegible scribble had been transformed into neat, orderly, very readable script—very convincing evidence that food and/or chemical allergies had been affecting her nervous system and causing poor penmanship.

Check your vision. If you wear glasses, periodically take them off and check your vision. I had one patient's eyesight return to normal after fasting. Food allergy had been affecting her sight.

Presenting Complaints: Hay fever, bronchitis, intermittent hyperactivity and hypoactivity, slurred speech, confusion. Patient was thought to be mentally retarded.

Dramatic Improvement in Penmanship While on a Rotary Diet After a Five-Day Fast

JANUARY 29, 1967	FEBRUARY 10, 1967	FEBRUARY 17, 1967
twenty twenty e	twenty twenty	twenty twenty
thirty thirty e	thirty thirty	thirty thirty
yf X fosty y forty	forty forty	forty forty
bffty bbfy bfty	bfty bfty	bfty bfty
siaty sixty s sil sity	sexty sixty	sixty sixty
seventy seventy	seventy seventy	seventy seventy
eighty eighty	eighty eighty	eighty eighty
ninty m ninty	ninty ninty	ninty ninty

BEFORE FASTING	5TH DAY of DIET	12TH DAY of DIET

Beef, eggs, and milk were the major offenders. When eliminated from the patient's diet, his mental cloud lifted and this sluggish-hyperactive child became alert and spoke clearly without pause or groping for words.

Other symptoms evoked during testing for milk and beef were nasal obstruction, coughing, pallor, restlessness, and irritability.

Diagnosis: ALLERGIC PSEUDO-RETARDATION.

After the Fast

Once you have fasted for five days, on the morning of the sixth day you will be ready to begin your series of food tests (and chemical tests—see chapter 6—if you have opted to test everything simultaneously). You should be comfortable, sleeping well, and your pulse should be below 80.

Quite possibly you have envisioned the first food you are to test as a one-food banquet. Don't count on it! Most people coming off a fast find their eyes are much bigger than their stomach, and while they may pile their plate high with the first food to be tested, they may not be able to eat much at all. What they usually learn, however, is that the food really tastes special. Carrots taste wonderfully like carrots, chicken tastes like farm-fresh chicken because the senses of smell and taste have become much more acute now that they are free of the chronic nasal congestion that is often a symptom of food allergy.

Many patients feel wonderful in many ways, better than they have felt in years. Your head should be clear, your mind alert, and you should be ready to experience and record the reactions that each food (and chemical) may bring on in your body and mind.

9
Controlling Your Food Allergies

Yours is not a hopeless case even if you reacted to many (or all) of the foods for which you tested yourself. The fact that you have allergies does not mean that you will have to serve a life sentence suffering from them. Now that you know some of the things to which you are allergic, you can begin your specific program to control the problems caused by them.

There is only one form of food allergy that is difficult to control; we call it fixed food allergy. With fixed allergy, no matter how many months you avoid an exposure to the food or beverage to which you are allergic, you will always have a reaction when you are reexposed. There are, however, other ways of controlling food allergy even of this type. If a neutralizing or relieving dose can be determined for a food, it may be used as a treatment to control the symptoms brought on by it. Neutralizing treatments can be given as a series of injections that are administered weekly or twice a week, or the neutralizing dose can be given at intervals sublingually (under the tongue) or taken before, during or after the meal that contains the food. Fixed food allergy can also be treated the way cases of hay fever are managed—by giving a series of injections of progressively increasing doses of a special form of the food extract to desensitize allergic individuals so that the food may be eaten with mild symptoms or no symptoms at all. Other ways to manage food allergy of this type include the use of nutritional supplements such as the vitamin and mineral insurance formula, high doses of vitamin C and B_6, and desiccated liver, as well as hydrochloric acid, sodium bicarbonate, and digestive enzymes.

Luckily, not all food allergies are fixed allergies; they are in the minority. Cyclic allergies constitute at least 50 percent of a patient's food allergies, and in some cases, as much as 90 percent. Cyclic allergies come and go, depending on the frequency of exposure and the quantity of food ingested. Reactions vary in intensity, sometimes severe, other times mild. If a number of potent allergy-provoking foods are eaten at the same time, the combined effects of several foods can be particularly severe. The nice thing about cyclic allergies is that if you give your system a rest period by avoiding the offending foods for a few weeks or months (this varies, too), you will acquire a tolerance for them. If you do not eat an offending food too often, the allergy remains dormant, and will remain so if tolerance is preserved by infrequent exposures, as when a Rotary Diversified Diet is followed.

What you have to do to find out which kind your allergies are is test yourself with the rest of the foods you eat, eliminate the foods to which you react for a period of six weeks, and then retest them periodically to see if you have regained your tolerance for any of them or if you have fixed allergies. I call this Diet for Life, Phase I. When you finally determine what forms of allergies you have, you can begin following Diet for Life, Phase II, an approach to diet planning that will help you avoid suddenly activating your dormant cyclic food allergies and prevent the development of new ones.

You *can* develop new allergies rather easily. Frequent exposure to a chemical or a food will decrease your resistance to it, and suddenly what did not bother you before, bothers you now. There is only one successful way to avoid developing new allergies, and that is the Diet for Life, along with good control over the chemical pollutants in your home, and, if possible, your work or school environment.

Something very interesting happened to one of my patients, a chemical and food allergic woman who smoked. I had urged her for months to give up smoking, and when she finally did, a large number of the foods to which she had been reacting no longer caused her any difficulties. Why? Because by giving up the toxic cigarette fumes to which she was chemically susceptible, she relieved herself of a tremendous biologic stress and her chemistry began to normalize.

Many of the foods to which she had been allergic because her system was continuously in a chemically toxic state no longer affected her. If you reduce your load of food allergies by following the Diet for Life, clean up your environment as recommended in chapter 6, and begin vitamin and mineral supplements as discussed in chapter 7, you will be working diligently toward a raised allergic threshold to many types of offenders. Once that happens, you are on the road to a controlled-allergy or allergy-free life.

Diet for Life, Phase I

The Diet for Life is really a two-phase operation. The first phase enables you to test the entire gamut of foods available for consumption to see just how many of them may be affecting your physical and mental health. The second phase makes it possible for you to start mixing and matching foods, and to begin to put more than one or two foods on your plate at a time. (Were you beginning to wonder if that would ever be possible?)

Since you have already tested yourself with one of the at-home tests, you already know some of the foods to which you are allergic. Fine. Now eliminate them from your diet for the next six weeks to enable your body to have a complete rest from reacting to them, and to build up a little tolerance to those allergies that are cyclic in nature.

The next step is to create your own diet plan to test all the foods you possibly can so you will have a complete knowledge of all the foods to which you are allergic. In order to organize your own test, you will have to design a schedule of foods that meets the following three criteria:

1. It doesn't include any of the foods to which you have an allergy.
2. It presents food on a schedule so that the same food does not appear more frequently than once in five days.
3. Foods from the same family do not appear more frequently than every other day.

Turn to the Biologic Classification of Foods on pages 241–244. You will probably find some unexpected surprises when you look over the botanists' and zoologists' classifications of foods according to their family relationships. For instance, under the heading Potato Family, you will see potato, tomato, eggplant, red pepper, cayenne, green pepper, and chili. Foods are now considered as members of biologic families (and this is a relatively new arrangement of foods) because in 1930 Dr. Warren Vaughan departed from the usual custom of classifying foods as fruits, nuts, vegetables, and meats and developed a more accurate system of classification based on similarity of their structure. Other workers have since refined and enlarged Vaughan's list.

The relationships between some of the foods is obvious to all. The similarities between oranges, tangerines, grapefruit, lemons, and limes are quite apparent. If you look carefully, cherries resemble nothing more closely than plums, of which they are a smaller version, and both are in the same family as peaches, apricots, and nectarines. The pits of peaches and apricots are very much like those of almonds, which belong to the family and really are not nuts. There is no such entity as a nut family —walnuts and pecans look very much alike and certainly are different in appearance from cashews and peanuts. Peanuts are part of the legume family and related to soybeans, peas, lima beans, and lentils, but to most people it comes as a surprise that licorice is also a member of this family. The cereal grains are members of the grass family, and it is easy to see how your neighbor's unkept lawn or a meadow where the grass has gone to seed looks very much like a wheat field, since they are all members of the same family. Sugarcane and bamboo are giant forms of grass, but buckwheat isn't a cereal at all—it happens to be a close relative of rhubarb. If you have ever remarked that beet tops look very much like spinach, you know why. Cauliflower really is a white variety of broccoli, or perhaps broccoli is green cauliflower. Brussels sprouts, in the same family (the mustard family), are just baby cabbages. Consider the similarities between an apple and a pear looked at end on—they are almost identical; so are zucchini and cucumbers—both members of the gourd family—when you slice them raw. In the same group, the similarities between pumpkin, cantaloupe, and honeydew are quite evident when you're busy scraping out seeds, and a careful inspection of watermelon will show that it too belongs to this family.

If you are allergic to one food within a family, there is an increased chance you will be allergic to another food or foods within that family. There is no way to be sure about your sensitivity to closely related foods unless you test all of them to see exactly what kind of reaction, if any, you have.

Since this is your period of testing, you do not have to be concerned about a balanced diet at this time. And do not worry about starting with the Vitamin and Mineral Insurance Formula and other nutritional supplements that were described in chapter 7. You will begin taking vitamins and minerals during the Diet for Life, Phase II. One step at a time—we do not want to complicate an already complex problem.

As with the other at-home tests presented throughout this book, you must obtain the most uncontaminated food available in your geographic area. This necessitates trips to the health food store or local organic farmers, or extremely careful purchases of foods in the local grocery store. The only prepared foods that have been found to be satisfactory are foods packaged in glass jars and frozen foods packaged in cardboard containers. Read the labels and make sure there are no preservatives or other foods in the products that might confuse your test results. I recommend health food store purchases because the food has been organically grown and meat comes from cows, chickens, sheep, and pigs that were fed on organically grown food in chemically free surroundings and not treated with antibiotics, growth stimulants, or tranquilizers.

Remember the alkaline salts in water if your symptoms become strong enough so that you do not want to wait for them to subside naturally: Mix 2 tablespoons of baking soda (sodium bicarbonate) with 1 tablespoon of potassium bicarbonate, and add a heaping teaspoon of this mixture to a large glass (12–16 ounces) of spring water. Aspirin-free Alka Seltzer Gold is also helpful and has a pleasanter taste. Take two successive doses of 1 tablet to a glass of water (total dose = 2 tablets in 16 ounces) in place of the alkaline salts. Milk of magnesia (unflavored) may be taken (2 to 4 tablespoons) for additional relief. If the symptoms are severe, you should try to empty your digestive tract and eliminate the food remaining in your system by taking a gentle but thorough laxative such as citrate of magnesia or phosphosoda (Fleet—unflavored) along with a sea salt or alkaline salts enema—use 2 level teaspoons of the salt(s) in a quart of lukewarm spring water.

Again, I caution those with kidney disease or heart disease that these sodium containing alkaline salts are not to be taken unless your physician says it is safe for you. Review all of the treatments for allergic reactions I have mentioned with your doctor and follow his advice. If it is available, oxygen for five to ten or fifteen minutes at a flow rate of six to seven liters a minute can be very helpful in relieving some reactions.

The spring water you drink must come from the spring in glass containers, which usually are available in five-gallon and half-gallon sizes. You want to eliminate or avoid as many chemical residues as possible, and plastic water bottles may contaminate the water they contain because they may gas out petroleum byproducts into the water itself. Be sure not to drink from plastic or waxed cups for the same reason.

Since you are now eliminating all those foods to which you have reacted in previous at-home tests, you have to begin to construct your own five-day diet.

Biologic Classification of Foods*

ANIMAL FOODS

Mollusks	Crayfish	*Fish*
Abalone	—	Sturgeon
—**	Lobster	Caviar
Mussel	—	—
Oyster	Shrimp	Anchovy
Scallop	—	Sardine
Clam	Squid	Herring
		Smelt
Crustaceans	*Amphibians*	Trout
Crab	Frog	Salmon

*Compiled by Dr. Theron G. Randolph. This is based on Vaughan's original classification as modified slightly by Ellis and confirmed for fish and seafood by the Shedd Aquarium, Chicago, and for plants by the Field Museum.
**Dashes between various groups of fish represent subdivisions, as there is some doubt as to the grouping of these fish. Authorities are not in complete agreement regarding the relationship of one group to another.

Whitefish
Chub
Shad
—
Eel
—
Carp
Sucker
Buffalo
—
Catfish
Bullhead
—
Pike
Pickerel
Muskellunge
—
Mullet
Barracuda
—
Mackerel
Tuna
Pompano
Bluefish
Butterfish
Harvestfish
Swordfish
—
Sunfish

Bass
Perch
Snapper
Croaker
Weakfish
Drum
Scup
Porgy
—
Flounder
Sole
Halibut
—
Rosefish
—
Codfish
Scrod
Haddock
Hake
Pollack
Cusk

Reptiles
Turtle

Mammals
Beef
  Veal
  Cow's milk

Butter
Cheese
Gelatin
Pork
  Ham
  Bacon
Goat
  Goat's milk
  Cheese
Mutton
  Lamb
Venison
Horse meat
Rabbit
Squirrel

Birds
Chicken
  Chicken eggs
Duck
  Duck eggs
Goose
  Goose eggs
Turkey
Guinea hen
Squab
Pheasant
Partridge
Grouse

PLANTS

Grains
Wheat
  Graham flour
  Gluten flour
  Bran
  Wheat germ
Rye
Barley
  Malt
Corn
  Cornstarch
  Corn oil
  Corn sugar

Corn syrup
Cerulose
Dextrose (Glucose)
Oats
Rice
Wild rice
Sorghum
Cane
  Cane sugar
  Molasses

Spurge Family
Tapioca

Arrowroot Family
Arrowroot

Arum Family
Taro
  Poi

Buckwheat Family
Buckwheat
Rhubarb

Potato Family
Potato

Tomato
Eggplant
Red pepper
  Cayenne
Green pepper
Chili

Composite Family
Leaf lettuce
Head lettuce
Endive
Escarole
Artichoke
Dandelion
Oyster plant
Chicory

Legumes
Navy bean
Kidney bean
Lima bean
String bean
Soy bean
  Soy bean oil
Lentil
Black-eyed peas
Pea
Peanut
  Peanut oil
Licorice
Acadia
Senna

Mustard Family
Mustard
Cabbage
Cauliflower
Broccoli
Brussels sprouts
Turnip
Rutabaga
Kale
Collard
Celery cabbage
Kohlrabi

Radish
Horseradish
Watercress

Gourd Family
Pumpkin
Squash
Cucumber
Cantaloupe
Muskmelon
Honeydew
Persian melon
Casaba
Watermelon

Lili Family
Asparagus
Onion
Garlic
Leek
Chive
Aloes

Goosefoot Family
Beet
  Beet sugar
Spinach
Swiss chard

Parsley Family
Parsley
Parsnip
Carrot
Celery
Celeriac
Caraway
Anise
Dill
Coriander
Fennel

Morning Glory Family
Sweet potato
Yam

Sunflower Family
Jerusalem artichoke
Sunflower seeds (oil)

Pomegranate Family
Pomegranate

Ebony Family
Persimmon

Rose Family
Raspberry
Blackberry
Loganberry
Youngberry
Dewberry
Strawberry

Banana Family
Banana

Apple Family
Apple
  Cider
  Vinegar
  Apple pectin
Pear
Quince
  Quince seed

Plum Family
Plum
  Prune
Cherry
Peach
Apricot
Nectarine
Almond

Laurel Family
Avocado
Cinnamon
Bay leaves

Olive Family
Green olive

Ripe olive
  Olive oil

Heath Family
Cranberry
Blueberry

Gooseberry Family
Gooseberry
Currant

Honeysuckle Family
Elderberry

Citrus Family
Orange
Grapefruit
Lemon
Lime
Tangerine
Kumquat

Pineapple Family
Pineapple

Papaw Family
Papaya

Grape Family
Grape
  Raisin
  Cream of tartar

Myrtle Family
Allspice
Cloves
Pimento
Paprika
Guava

Mint Family
Mint
Peppermint
Spearmint
Thyme

Sage
Marjoram
Savory

Pepper Family
Black pepper

Nutmeg Family
Nutmeg

Ginger Family
Ginger
Turmeric
Cardamon

Pine Family
Juniper

Orchid Family
Vanilla

Madder Family
Coffee

Tea Family
Tea

Pedalium Family
Sesame seeds
Sesame oil

Mallow Family
Okra (Gumbo)
Cottonseed

Stercula Family
Cocoa
  Chocolate

Birch Family
Filbert
Hazelnut
Oil of birch
  (Wintergreen)

Mulberry Family
Mulberry
Fig
Hop
Breadfruit

Maple Family
Maple syrup
  Maple sugar

Palm Family
Coconut
Date
Sago

Lecythis Family
Brazil nut

Poppy Family
Poppy seed

Walnut Family
English walnut
Black walnut
Butternut
Hickory nut
Pecan

Cashew Family
Cashew
Pistachio
Mango

Beech Family
Chestnut

Fungi
Mushroom
Yeast

Miscellaneous
Honey

Sample 5-Day Diet for Those Who Are Allergic to Beef, Milk, Wheat, Chicken, Eggs, Tomato, and Lettuce

DAY	BREAKFAST	LUNCH	DINNER
#1	Apple or pear	Squash or pumpkin	Lamb or goat
#2	Orange or grapefruit	Lima beans or peas	Salmon or trout
#3	Pineapple	Carrot or celery	Duck, goose, or turkey
#4	Cantaloupe or honeydew	Sweet potato or yam	Lobster, shrimp, or crab
#5	Banana	Cabbage, broccoli, or beet	Pork

The key to this diet and to the diet you create is that once you eat a particular food, you do not eat it again in any form for at least five days. And make sure not to eat any members of the same family more frequently than every other day.

Once you have completed the first five days on the Rotary Diversified Diet, you can begin substituting new foods in place of the ones tested.

Note, of course, that there is no beef, milk, wheat, chicken, egg, tomato, or lettuce in this sample diet. However, after about six to eight weeks, the person allergic to these foods can begin to reintroduce them one at a time to see if tolerance has been regained during this interval, keeping in mind that it may take as long as three, four, or six months for some foods. You must learn if each food allergy is fixed or cyclic. If it is fixed, the food cannot be eaten without producing allergic symptoms, unless there is special treatment to reduce or block these symptoms. If it is cyclic, the food can be eaten as long as exposures to it are placed far enough apart so that the allergy does not become reactivated. Each reader will discover his or her own allergies and have to develop an individual five-day rotation diet. (By the way, a five-day rotation is the minimum rotation I recommend for foods, but, at times, seven, ten, twelve, or fourteen days are required by some of my patients.)

As you progress through all the foods you want to test, carefully observe all of your reactions and record all of the important information gathered from your food-ingestion tests. Review your notes in detail, making additions of foods that you have not yet tested and substituting foods for those to which you find you are allergic, until you have tested and retested them all. If you want to test for allergies to spices, simply put a spice on a test-negative food—red pepper on shrimp, garlic on lamb, cinnamon on apple, mustard on beef, paprika on chicken, and so forth. If you want to test an oil, use it on or with a food to which you know you are not allergic.

Soon you will have a list of foods you can eat and lists of foods you know you are slightly or very allergic to. But remember, the key to successful testing is to separate the foods within the same families by every other day, whether you react to them or not, and not to repeat any food for at least five days.

After you have completed testing, you move on to Diet for Life, Phase II.

Diet for Life, Phase II

I know there is nothing that some of you would probably rather do than sit down right now and have a huge plate of lasagna or a heaping dish of your favorite ice cream or a plate filled with different vegetables and gravy-covered meat. But you cannot do it at this time. Reintroduction of food mixtures or several foods per meal to your diet is something that has to be approached with caution. You must always be in control of the entire situation so you can learn as much as possible about the way foods affect your health.

Because you are an allergic person, you have to live with certain irrefutable facts: Although you now have your list of foods to which you are not allergic and are psychologically ready to put a few of them on the plate at the same time, you must understand that if you combine foods to which you have had no reaction during testing, you could have an allergic reaction. This happens because the minor allergy you have to these foods was not detected during testing, but when you eat them together, you react to their combined effects. This does not present an impossible situation, although it is one more indication of just how complex the problems can be. What you have to do in Diet for Life, Phase II is put together two foods that you have eaten from four to six times in rotation and seemed to tolerate, and observe the effects of the combined foods. Then you may try combinations of three foods to observe their effect. It is essential that you keep detailed notes because the situation will become so confusing without them that you will be completely lost. Without having notes to which to refer, a complex problem like multiple food allergies will become much more difficult than it has to be.

Within a matter of days or weeks you will have a list of foods that are compatible with each other and may be combined to give you two- and three-food meals! I realize that some readers may think that I am asking a great deal of them, but there are very few shortcuts that can be taken when one is trying to correct many years of physical and mental illness by controlling its cause and avoiding the use of medications. Life will be much simpler in the future when we learn how to prevent allergies or how to treat them by employing biologically and physiologically sound measures that are effective and simple. At the present time, dietary and environmental control in conjunction with desensitizing treatments and nutritional therapy are, in my opinion, preferable to the use of drugs, and other forms of treatment which often have many undesirable side effects.

Another interesting aspect of food allergy is that for years allergists have known that some children can not handle pasteurized milk, which has little heating, but can drink evaporated milk, which receives much more heating during its preparation. A young boy in my practice who had no symptoms when he drank milk at home could not drink the milk that was served at school. The milk supply that was served at home was raw milk obtained from a neighbor's dairy farm, and the milk at school was pasteurized. Therefore, you may react to a food in its cooked form but not its uncooked form, or vice versa. So take the list of foods to which you are allergic and try cooking them if you usually eat them raw, or try eating them raw if you normally eat them cooked. Some foods will be tolerated if they are stir-fried in an oil to which you do not react. By approaching allergy systematically in a commonsense manner, you will be able to deal with many problems.

A Transition in Thinking

By this time you may have gotten the impression that the rotation of foods on a five-, seven-, or ten-day schedule is going to be your way of life for some time. It is—at least until the problems of allergy are solved by the biochemists and physiologists. Good food and pure water are a vital necessity. Nutritional supplementation with vitamins and minerals, desensitizing treatments and comprehensive environmental control are also essential parts of your health picture. It is only by this overall approach that man is going to begin to recover and undo some of the damage he has done to himself and his environment. And I must add that promising developments in biofeedback and kinesiology will also have an important role in the total health picture.

You have to make a choice. You can live your life half-well (as many people do), or you can really make a concerted effort to achieve optimal health by changing your way of thinking and your style of living. With foods, in particular, a different point of view is necessary. You must understand that eating a meal was not designed by nature to be a great social event or a gourmet gastronomic delight. Eating really is the intake of essential energy and building materials to sustain life, to promote growth, and to repair the body. The habits of a lifetime may have to be changed when it comes to the foods you can eat and still remain free from serious forms of bodywide allergic symptoms.

Like you, I have enjoyed and deeply appreciated the many pleasures one gets from a tasty and attractive meal in the presence of those whom one likes, loves, or is just getting to know. It can be a frustrating experience to think about the aroma and relive the wonderful taste of favorite foods that are now off limits, but some of this will have to be sacrificed in order for you to get well and stay well. Your health must come first. A well-known and widely respected colleague told me that it just was not worth it for him to eat wheat or corn and get a nagging headache and be unable to concentrate or think clearly for the

next day or two. These two foods would make it impossible for
him to take care of his patients because of their severe effect on
his nervous system. He refused to live in confusion or be unable
to function. The price he had to pay for enjoying them was too
high for him. And when you know the facts in your own particular case, the decision will not really be a difficult one for you to
make either.

10

What the Future Holds

Doctors' Resistance

Doctors are in conflict, and I understand it well. I experienced it, too, as did all my colleagues at one time or another prior to becoming involved in bio-ecologic medicine. That allergy and chemical susceptibility could constitute from 50 to 80 percent of the daily medical practice of many doctors (and essentially that is the correct inference other physicians draw from our published works) comes as a terrible shock to them because it undermines much of the foundation upon which their medical practice is based. At first, almost everything in which they ever believed in medicine seems to be at stake if they were to accept our approach to medicine. In a sense, they really do have to relearn medicine, acquire a new perspective, and see many diseases in a different light. It is not easy for physicians to relinquish their beliefs and methods overnight; for some it may be impossible.

It is especially difficult for doctors to accept our discovery that allergy is at the core of so much mental and physical illness. Allergy was barely even mentioned in medical school, and those who did receive a smattering of information about allergy certainly were not taught anything like what my colleagues and I have been reporting as major discoveries of the greatest importance. Now, all of a sudden, we are telling these doctors that for years they have been on the wrong track; that, in effect, if they do not take the time to educate themselves about our findings, they will be practicing an inferior brand of medicine.

And that is exactly what we are saying. We've said it as nicely and professionally as possible through lectures around the world, through many articles published in medical literature, and by means of one-to-one conversations, but the wall of resistance to change has been an extremely difficult one to break through.

This "turning a deaf ear" is something my colleagues and I encounter constantly. Sometimes it takes firsthand evidence before my work and the work of my colleagues is given credence. For example, after a physician friend of mine confided to me that on many days around three or four o'clock in the afternoon he wished that all his patients would go home and leave him alone because he felt so terribly tired, I tested him and made him very sleepy, proving that his afternoon fatigue was due to the milk he put in his coffee at lunchtime and in ice cream he usually had for dessert after lunch. His chronic abdominal distress and bloating were also eliminated when I found that ham, bacon and sausage (pork) were the culprits he was exposed to daily at breakfast.

His wife had been under the care of one of our community's highly respected physicians who had diagnosed her problem as spastic colitis due to emotional causes. She was taking a number of medications and had followed various "colitis" diets for eight years. After five days of therapeutic fasting under my supervision, her condition cleared up completely for the first time. She no longer had abdominal pain or diarrhea and was not passing any more gas or bloody mucus.

I started her on a diagnostic rotary diet to determine the foods to which she might be allergic. She was fine until she took her test for coffee allergy. Within minutes after drinking a cup of black coffee, all the usual symptoms of her assumed "emotional" illness were reproduced in a very convincing manner.

She was a particularly interesting case of food allergy because she was one of the very few patients I have ever seen where a *single* factor was identified as being the only cause of a long-term illness. Management of this case was incredibly simple. She was permitted to eat all of the foods she had eaten in the past, but on a rotary basis, and she had to eliminate coffee. *There was no further need for any medication because she did not have any symptoms after the cause of her disorder was iden-tified and eliminated.* For the first time in many years, her gastrointestional tract began to function properly and absorb foods normally. She gained a badly needed sixteen pounds, which brought her up to her proper weight after being pain-fully thin.

To me, one of the outstanding aspects of her case (aside from the fact that it is most unusual to have a single food offender and achieve a cure by such a simple measure as eliminating coffee) concerns the attitude of the physician who had been treating this woman with partially effective supressive medications for *eight years.* When my colleague told him about the miraculous transformation in his wife's health and the methods by which I established the diagnosis of colitis due to coffee allergy, the doctor did not make any comment. Not a single word. Nor did he ever get in touch with me to discuss my management of this case and the likely possibility that other patients under his care might have similar problems. To date, and this goes back at least six years, he has never referred a single case to me. *He had been treating this woman for eight years, and I "cured" her without drugs in five days.* Was he embarrassed? Stubborn? Afraid to be different from his local peers? Not interested in learning about another way to do things, natural and nondrug, and gaining additional skills? This is a classic example of human nature ver-sus scientific/medical progress.

It is the rare psychiatrist who ever appreciated being told that his patient's nervousness, schizophrenia, depression, cata-tonia, autism, anxiety, violence might be a form of bio-ecologic illness due to a reversible kind of nervous system allergy to something present in his diet, water, or environment, and not the result of some deep-seated psychic trauma having its roots in childhood. Few of my fellow allergists have ever welcomed the knowledge that many of the tests they currently employ are not accurate and the professional care they are rendering in many cases is at a level considerably below what they could accomplish if they were to employ our more accurate and com-prehensive diagnostic and therapeutic methods. Few internists have ever said, "Dr. Mandell, this is tremendously exciting," when told that patients' severe itching, headaches, arthritis, fatigue, bladder problems, depression, intestinal, or gastric complaints might be due to something as simple as an allergy to milk, wheat, beef, eggs, or some other commonly eaten food, even though the internist will readily admit he could not find a reason for his patients' complaints after a careful examination and extensive laboratory tests. Instead of ruling out the possibility of bio-ecologic illness being present, he will relieve himself of this responsibility and send such patients to a psychiatrist.

A friend of mine sent me a copy of a letter written to the editor of one of the pediatric journals in which the physician stated that she had observed in her practice that she was doing more follow-up urine examinations for urinary tract infections in allergic children than she was doing in the general population of her practice. She inquired of the editor of the journal whether there might be some association between allergy and such infections and symptoms of infection. Because of my experience in this area, I sent a four-page letter to the editor in which I stated that urinary tract disorders on an allergic basis were quite common. I wrote that I had seen approximately thirty-five such patients in whom testing with extracts in the office produced typical symptoms of frequent, urgent, uncomfortable urination and that most of these tests had been confirmed by ingestion tests at home following Dr. Rinkel's feeding test technique, and I described a number of cases.

I received a letter from the editor thanking me for sending the information but stating he felt he could not publish it because I was only giving *anecdotal* information. In other words, I was only giving him my observations and giving him case reports, but I had no controls and therefore my material was not appropriate for this particular pediatric journal. I wrote back to him stating that I felt he should give lower urinary tract allergy serious consideration since it not only imitated infection but in my experience it could lead to infection and was also responsible for quite a few cases of bedwetting and bladder discomfort. In his second letter, he replied that he had presented all my information to several pediatricians who had considerable clinical experience and none of them had ever read about it or heard about it or believed that they had ever seen such a case and therefore the editor still could not publish it. Once again I wrote and stated that the fact that they had not read about it was because no one had yet had their observations published and this is what I was seeking to do, not as a formal paper but merely as an informative letter to the editor indicating that lower urinary tract allergy was indeed a reality which I and a number of my colleagues had seen frequently.

I also mentioned to him that Dr. Norborne Powell, professor of urology at Baylor University, one of the leading medical schools in Texas, had recently informed me that those patients who were managed medically and failed to respond to his treatment were then treated surgically, and the majority of them were surgical failures as well. When he became aware of the existence of lower urinary tract allergy, he tested approximately sixty of these patients whose medical and surgical treatment had failed, and was able to demonstrate the presence of urinary tract allergy in all but a very small number of this series of cases. I also indicated that a former president of the American College of Allergists (Dr. John McGovern) had written a paper with Dr. Powell in which they discussed the diagnosis and treatment of lower urinary tract allergy due to pollens, dusts, and molds. Dr. Powell and Dr. McGovern's observations published in the *Annals of Allergy* were ignored as well as my letter. In effect, the editor of a major pediatric journal refused to expose his readers to a body of very important new medical information because it was unfamiliar to him and several other pediatricians who knew nothing about bladder allergy in children.

This type of thinking certainly was not limited to the editor of one of the leading pediatric journals. Dr. Powell and I got the same response from the American Urologic Association, which publishes the *Journal of Urology* and is the professional organization to which the country's leading urologists belong. Dr. Powell and I had applied to present our combined findings to the annual meeting of the urinary tract specialists; we wanted to give preliminary reports on the importance of allergy in these conditions and how they had been previously unrecognized and overlooked as a very important aspect of a urologic practice.

This occurred at least five years ago and it is not possible for me to estimate how much unnecessary pain, loss of time, unnecessary medication, and avoidable surgery have occurred because of this modern medical tragedy. And I wonder how many thousands upon thousands of wasted hours have been spent in the psychiatrist's office in a useless attempt to determine the nonexistent emotional factors that were incorrectly assumed to have led to lower abdominal pains, urinary frequency and urgency as well as genital discomfort because the urologists could find absolutely nothing wrong with the patients and concluded that the unrecognized allergies must be emotional disorders. We have to discard the tremendous influence of psychiatric concepts that are postulated as explanations for disease. We have to get rid of most of it—not all of it. Neither my colleagues nor I would ever deny the importance of emotional factors or unconscious mental processes; but just because they exist we can no longer blame them for everything that wasn't previously understood. The sense of tragedy and overwhelming frustration that we feel is based on the realization that our knowledge could be applied beneficially and those who should have this knowledge, unfortunately, do not possess it.

I was at a staff meeting at the department of medicine in our local hospital recently among physicians with whom I have always maintained cordial relations. I listened carefully and respectfully as these highly trained and conscientious physicians thoroughly discussed a particular patient's complex medical problem. As they reviewed the situation, it was obvious that these clinicians had individually and collectively accumulated a massive amount of knowledge and experience. There was no question that they were well acquainted with the variations within many diseases and the latest techniques by which to diagnose them. They were familiar with all of the currently employed medications for the treatment of different illnesses and they demonstrated a wealth of information regarding the drugs of choice (the safest drugs that would be least likely to cause harmful side effects) and the drugs that would be incompatible with each other. These concerned physicians (whose work load is often monumental) put in many hours of effort every working day to help their patients, and they spend much additional time in order to keep up with medical progress. (I see their cars going in and out of the hospital parking lot across the street from my office late at night and early in the morning.) And yet, as I followed their discussion, I felt that I was present in a real and yet unreal, almost schizophrenic, kind of atmosphere. I was in what seemed to be a familiar and yet somehow strange place where everybody's orientation was confused and I sensed that the entire conference was going in the wrong direction.

They spent a considerable amount of time discussing the many ways in which the disease could progress and the various medications that could be administered etc., etc. . . ., but with all the combined years of clinical experience upon which to draw and all the excellent intellects we had working together during that staff conference, no one was asking what I believe are among some of the most important questions physicians can ask:

Why is this patient sick?
What specifically is making him ill?
Can we help his natural defense mechanisms combat this disorder?
Is there anything we can do to build up a healthier body to prevent an illness of this kind?
Shall we make some changes in his diet or his environment?

Not a single physician said:

I don't want to suppress these symptoms with long-term medications that may cause undesirable side effects.
I would like to find out why he is so sick and if I knew the factors that were causing his illness, perhaps I could control it and he would not need any drug treatment at all.

I felt as though I were a stranger visiting from another planet or in some strange kind of world. Something terribly wrong was happening and nobody in the conference room seemed to realize that a very important piece of the puzzle was missing, and that they had forgotten to look for the *cause* of the patient's problem.

The knowledge that commonly eaten foods, beverages (including water), numerous environmental chemicals, and dusts, molds, pollens, and animal danders can be the underlying cause of important types of physical and mental illness is one of the most important breakthroughs in modern medicine. And it comes as a big shock to most traditionally trained doctors to be told that there is something very special that we bio-ecologists know that they do not know and this knowledge is going to change the course of medicine forever. The physicians who are deeply involved in allergy, addiction, ecology, and nutrition as major underlying factors in the cause of many of mankind's serious health problems are not a group of wild-eyed young antiestablishment physicians. On the contrary, most of us became interested in biology and ecology after many years of practicing in different specialties of traditional medicine. Despite our certification as medical experts by the various specialty boards, we were often confronted with, and frustrated by, gaping holes in our knowledge that demanded answers. So we began to look for the reasons why our patients were ill and why our treatments were not always successful. Together, we found many of the answers in various aspects of allergy, in nutrition, and in the effects of our increasingly polluted environment which makes it difficult, if not impossible, for human beings to be really healthy. And, over a period of time, we developed an effective but rather complex commonsense system by which we could help our patients and by which they could help themselves without the use of drugs. It was, and is, a very exciting time in medical history for one to be a physician.

An Open Invitation to Other Doctors

I can almost guarantee any open-minded physicians who sincerely want to help their patients that after spending three to five full days with us at the Alan Mandell Center for Bio-Ecologic Disease, they will leave my office with a totally new outlook on medicine. They probably will be eager to get back to their practices and reevaluate some of their current problem cases and recall those patients which they will realize did not have to be given up on or maintained on programs of symptom-suppressing medications. The diagnostically useful information gained during my consultations with a group of unselected patients will be clinical revelations that will appeal to their sense of logic. Testing will clearly demonstrate the importance of allergy, addiction, and chemical susceptibility in physical and mental illness—and in many instances, the roles of these factors will be dramatically highlighted as the patients react to their tests. The not-too-difficult-to-achieve near miracles that often take place here at the Center can be overwhelming to the guest observer at first as some of our patients under treatment often eloquently describe their long search for health. The orientation and thrust of the medical practices of these visiting physicians will be changed forever if they have the courage to practice what they have observed here and now know to be true.

For over ten years, I have had an "open door" policy regarding professional visitors at the Center. Physicians have always been welcome to visit and observe my work at any time without a formal invitation. They may come to the Center to see what we do, talk with us, talk with patients, watch testing, and see results. "Within the reasonable limitations of time and space, all who are qualified for admission to the office as visitor-observers are welcome at any time without any formal invitation; they will be accommodated to the best of our ability. Chance alone will determine the activities in progress at the time of the visit, but with the patient's consent, the consultation room, testing rooms and office records are open for observation and study. Any staff member or consenting patient may be interviewed privately as circumstances permit.

"We do not claim to have all the answers to the many problems of reversible functional types of physical and mental illness but we welcome the opportunity to share what we have learned with all who are interested and hope to have them join us in participating in this most promising area of medicine."*

---

*Marshall Mandell, "Ecologic Concepts and Techniques: Their Impact on an Allergist and His Practice." In L. Dickey, ed., *Clinical Ecology* (Springfield, Ill.: Charles C. Thomas, 1976), p. 627.

How to Find a Doctor

It is not going to be easy. At present, there is only a small group of self-taught physicians who are sufficiently familiar with allergy, clinical ecology, nutrition, orthomolecular psychiatry, and preventive medicine, to be able to help some of the most difficult medical problems that are brought to our attention.

We are self-taught because there is no medical school in this country whose board of trustees and senior faculty members have the vision, knowledge, or perhaps, the simple courage to give its students or graduate students a broad-based, holistic perspective of human health and disease. To be self-taught is not an easy task because there are many people with whom to confer, meetings to attend, places to visit, techniques to learn, literature to read—and at the same time one has a practice to which to attend, family obligations, and a need for some time off for just living and enjoying life.

So it is not going to be easy to find a doctor who really understands bio-ecologic illness and allergy, but a good starting point in your search for an ecologically oriented physician would be to see if any members of the Society for Clinical Ecology reside in your general vicinity. The Society was established in 1965 by a group of concerned physicians and allergists (myself included) because of the serious differences in opinion regarding the directions that we and the national allergy societies wished to follow. At the present time there are more than two hundred members in our organization. The majority of them are medical doctors, but there also is a small group of Ph.D.'s in chemistry, nutrition and psychology, engineers, and laymen who are interested in many facets of ecology, especially ecologic illness. For information regarding the Society for Clinical Ecology, write to Robert Collier, MD, 4045 Wadsworth Blvd., Wheat Ridge, Colorado 80033. He should be able to give you the name of a physician in your general area who might be able to help you.

I want to emphasize that not all of the physicians in the Society for Clinical Ecology are as deeply involved in all phases of clinical ecology as some of my colleagues and I who were the founders of the Society. Our new associate physicians are learning quickly, and by joining us they show that they have open minds and an interest in gaining a more comprehensive knowledge of bio-ecologic illness and allergy. To facilitate finding one of the physicians who has a broad knowledge of the subject based on experience and who is totally committed to this work, I have developed a list of questions for you to use when interviewing your prospective doctor or discussing him with a member of his staff. Save yourself an initial visit by asking the doctor or his appointed representative (nurse or receptionist usually) the following questions over the phone.*

1. *Is he a Fellow or Associate Fellow of the Society for Clinical Ecology?* Membership in various organizations will not guarantee that we do not have a chronic joiner who wants to cover his walls with membership certificates, but at least you have an indication that he was interested. Ask how many meetings he has been to and when he went last. After all, he could pay a few dollars and become an associate member and then drop out and never pay any dues or never go to any meetings—but he would have a membership certificate that no authority could come and take off his wall. Although it might be impressive, it also could be meaningless.

2. *How long has he practiced in his field?* Most clinical ecologists with a thorough knowledge of bio-ecologic illness are not young doctors. Quite the contrary. Most physicians specializing in our field are those doctors who spent many long years in traditional practice before they realized the limitations of those practices and became clinical ecologists. That is not to say that

---

*You must realize that a physician may not have time to speak at length on the telephone. He or she cannot usually spend all the time it would take to give you all the answers you would like to have. A busy physician could be tied up for hours by answering questions of prospective patients or their relatives, and this would require too much of his or her productive time. In my office, the secretaries take care of over 90 percent of these calls, and mail a package of information and reprints of some of my papers or articles concerning my work to those who request information. If there are any medical questions that my secretaries or staff nurses cannot answer, they discuss the matter with me as soon as it is convenient and telephone or mail the requested information. In very complex situations we arrange, when appropriate, a previsit telephone consultation with me by appointment.

a young doctor couldn't be a clinical ecologist. It is just highly unlikely because no medical school teaches the subject of bio-ecologic illness and allergy, and most of my colleagues are self-taught, which takes many years.

3. *Does he perform "provocative" tests by ingestion, inhalation, injections or extracts under the tongue?* If he doesn't, then he is not familiar with (or hasn't accepted) the new, proven techniques for determining whether a patient is truly allergic. If he relies on the old methods of skin testing he is not up-to-date in bio-ecologic medicine.

4. *With whom has he studied, and for how long?* This is important. There are very few bio-ecologic physicians around. (The vast majority of the doctors in practice are traditional doctors who still believe in the old ways.) If a doctor can't tell you who Drs. Theron Randolph, Herbert Rinkel, and Carleton Lee are and can't say he endorses their work, then he isn't one of us. He certainly should be familiar with my work and, in general, agree with the fundamental concepts presented in this book.

5. *Has he presented and/or published any papers on the subject of bio-ecologic illness and allergy?* If he has, this certainly shows an active interest in the subject. Ask him to send you a few reprints of his published papers.

I will tell you right now that many doctors and their staffs will resent this kind of simple inquiry. They are not used to it. Most doctors are used to having patients arrive by referral from other doctors or patients and rarely does the patient become the interviewer. Those doctors, however, who are involved in bio-ecologic illness and allergy will be more than willing to have their secretaries or nurses talk with you about the office's area of interest and expertise. At the least, their staff will be able to give you some indicative answers to your questions that will help you determine whether or not the doctor is the one for you. But telephone first. There is no reason to pay an "initial visit" fee only to find out that there won't be a second visit.

Also, I want to emphasize that although a doctor may not employ all of our techniques, he certainly should be aware of them and respect them. No physician is competent in every aspect of medicine. For instance I have not yet employed chiropractic kinesiology, but I am certain that it will benefit many patients. I am not employing biofeedback at the Center yet, but I recognize that it is important and plan to study it as soon as I have the opportunity to do so in sufficient depth to incorporate it in my practice. I am not skilled in the diagnosis of temperomandibular joint (TMJ) dysfunction but I recognize its importance. The area of visualmotor integration (VMI) is important in pediatrics and must be utilized much more often.

If a doctor does not practice clinical ecology, he should at least have an acquaintance with our work, and if not an authority on the subject, at least be open-minded about it so he can refer patients elsewhere if they need it. With the knowledge explosion in science no doctor can be a complete physician. He cannot serve his patients' best interests unless he recognizes his limitations and is willing to consult with others who have skills with which he is not totally familiar or in which he is not highly proficient. We recognize that we don't know everything, that our skills are not without limits, too.

What about Hospitals?

At the present time there are probably fewer than fifty beds available in hospitals in the entire United States for extensive testing for bio-ecologic disease by means of comprehensive environmental control, and this totally inadequate number of beds is constantly being threatened. The reason there are so few beds available is that the individuals who could make such facilities available in local hospitals—or at least in regional hospitals—do not realize how important and how common these diseases are. Also, physicians who practice bio-ecological medicine are few in number and, in most instances, widely separated geographically. Their patients often come from several hundred miles away, and the local doctors (and the hospital administration and staff) frequently resent, resist, and reject the elective admission of out-of-town patients because most of these hospitals are community-supported local hospitals designed to serve the community, not outsiders. This is certainly an understandable attitude when bed shortage (which is prevalent in most local hospitals) is considered objectively.

Teaching hospitals affiliated with medical schools and special facilities for respiratory diseases, mental illness, alcoholism, and the various types of chronic disorders are the most logical institutions in which patients suffering from advanced forms of environmental allergies that require a totally controlled chemically unpolluted environment and constant care should be treated. However, at the present time there is still very little or no recognition of the importance of environmental factors as they are appreciated by clinical ecologists in any teaching hospitals. Even if there are physicians in the area who practice the bio-ecologically oriented type of medicine in which my colleagues and I specialize, there is a 99.9 percent chance that the local medical community will not readily accept the physician whose concept of what causes mental and physical ailments is different from theirs. Sometimes, however, private hospitals will allow a patient to be admitted for fasting and treatment, and occasionally a local public hospital will make an "exception to the rule."

The Promise of Bio-Ecologic Medicine

The discoveries we have made over the past twenty-five years have shed new light on diseases and have opened a whole new field of medicine to explore.

CANCER TREATMENTS

Carleton Lee, MD, St. Joseph, Missouri, the physician who discovered the neutralizing techniques that enabled him to stop a patient's allergic reaction, has, with the help of a few of our colleagues, become involved in conducting some very exciting studies on a small group of cancer patients suffering from the late stages of inoperable malignancies. Severe pain has been controlled in some cancer patients by Lee's neutralizing technique, which employs different concentrations of extracts prepared from surgical specimens of each patient's own tumor. In several instances, the use of narcotics was completely eliminated and the mental cloud associated with the use of large doses of narcotics was removed. Not only was the pain controlled, but in some cases there was a definite regression in the size of the remaining tumor mass and a prolongation of life.

Dr. X,* an inspired student of Dr. Lee's, recently told me about a middle-aged woman who had already been operated on for cancer in her left breast. Unfortunately, several other malignant tumors of the same type later appeared in her right breast. Dr. X was able to obtain a specimen of the cancer that had been removed during the first operation; he prepared a tumor extract which he processed in a blender and then prepared a series of dilutions of this material to observe any possible effects that might be obtained by administering the extract to the patient.

We owe a great debt of gratitude to this courageous lady patient for her willingness to participate in this study by Dr. X. Future generations of women, and perhaps other patients with other forms of cancer, may some day owe their lives to her. Although there is still a great deal that must be done in the direction so brilliantly pointed out by Dr. X, several important facts emerged:

1. A specific dilution of the breast tumor extract injected into the patient's arm caused immediate swelling and increased pain within a few minutes in the tumors present in the remaining breast just under the skin. In fact, the increase in the size of the cancer was plainly visible.
2. Another dilution of her breast cancer extract promptly relieved the pain in the tumor and reduced the swelling caused by the provoking dose of her breast cancer extract.
3. Dr. X was able to relieve both pain and swelling of the breast cancer in this woman by "neutralizing" injections of tumor tissue extract prepared from a surgical specimen of her original malignancy.

Dr. Lee told me about a patient with cancer of the prostate who had been receiving chemotherapy without any relief of

*This doctor, a close friend of mine and a highly respected colleague, wishes to remain anonymous until more of his studies are completed.

pain from the treatment. He was going downhill rapidly and his personal physician asked Dr. Lee if he could help. No specimen of the patient's cancer tissue was available in this case, and Dr. Lee used an extract he had prepared from a prostate cancer in another patient. Under Dr. Lee's supervision, this patient's allergist (who practiced clinical ecology) arrived at a neutralizing dose of the prostate cancer extract and brought about complete relief from pain without any narcotics' being required as they had been until that time. In addition, within two weeks this patient's severe anemia, which had been present for a considerable time, was greatly improved, and he was able to return to work. He remained comfortable with neutralizing treatments for a period of one year, requiring no painkiller whatsoever.

A second case related to me by Dr. Lee was that of a fifty-year-old man in the last stages of multiple melanoma spread throughout his body and causing severe pain. The patient had been treated with heavy doses of narcotics in the hospital because the pain made it impossible for him to sleep. This man's surgeon knew Dr. Lee well. At the surgeon's suggestion Dr. Lee prepared a series of dilutions of biopsy material from a tumor mass that had invaded the patient's muscle. When the neutralizing dose was determined, the patient was relieved of pain for over a year, and he would otherwise have suffered intensely. In addition, the patient's mental cloud from pain-killing drugs lifted; there was no further need for any mind-dulling narcotics. After neutralizing, he was able to sleep well, became able to leave the hospital, and continued to work until the last two months of his life.

A third patient was a forty-six-year-old woman who had a breast cancer removed one and a half years prior to being seen by Dr. Lee. She came to him for hay fever and asthma and incidentally mentioned that she had a severe tenderness in the area of her breastbone. The tenderness was of such intensity that she had to wear a very loose blouse to reduce the painful pressure of her clothing in this area. After examining the area, Dr. Lee referred her back to her surgeon, who performed a biopsy and confirmed the fact that the breast cancer had spread to the skeleton. Two weeks later, an area of tenderness was noted in the back of her head toward the base of the skull (occipital region) and a biopsy specimen was taken which confirmed that this, too, was a metastatic cancer.

The consensus at that time was that this woman had about six weeks to live. A series of dilutions were prepared for neutralizing treatments from the specimen taken from her skull, and the local pain in the breastbone (sternum) and her skull was controlled. This pain was described as being severe in intensity. The neutralizing dose was given every four days as needed to control pain. The patient's radiologist was surprised to note on her X-rays that the area invaded by tumor actually was healing and new bone was forming.

With neutralizing treatment, this woman, who had been given six weeks to live, did live comfortably for two and one-half years. Dr. Lee and I share the belief that we do indeed have something important here that is not well understood but certainly seems to have much promise. More studies must be done to understand the temporary relief of pain that has been obtained. His question was, "What did I do that led to the regeneration of new bone and healing at the sites of a metastatic cancer?"

I wish to make it clear to the reader that the evidence to date is very limited in terms of numbers of cases, but we really cannot afford to ignore observations of this nature. Although the fundamental mechanism of neutralizing technique is not fully known at present, it is indeed unfortunate that it should be ignored or rejected by members of the medical establishment. The limited number of patients suffering from cancer who have cooperated in such studies were ones whose disease was so far gone that it was felt that they could not be harmed by such a procedure and that they really had nothing to lose. This work must be continued and extended in great depth because it appears to hold considerable promise. In some cases, it is quite possible that neutralization treatment may be as effective as or more effective than chemotherapy radiation therapy, extensive surgery, or the use of high doses of narcotics.

DYSMENORRHEA (PAINFUL MENSTRUAL PERIODS)

Dr. Joseph Miller, of Mobile, Alabama, has also employed the neutralizing technique with women suffering from excruciatingly painful menstrual periods. By giving more than a hundred women with a history of painful menstrual periods neutralizing doses of progesterone, the hormone that builds up shortly before the menstrual period begins, he has been able to reduce or eliminate the pain associated with menstrual periods as well as attendant tension, hives, migraine headache, fluid retention, and asthma. A group of gynecologists in Texas to whom he taught his technique were able to help over a hundred more women also suffering from dysmenorrhea. With the help of neutralization, problems related to menstrual flow have been controlled; this involves women who have had a scant menstrual flow as well as women with excessive menstrual flow.

Women with a tendency to have an acute flare-up of acne coincidental with their menses have had dramatic improvement in their skin condition. Although the acne outbreak appears in the skin just before or during menses, the acne may persist for weeks thereafter; this phase of skin eruption has been controlled, too. The other female hormone, estrogen, has also been employed in neutralizing treatments. To date, there have been twenty cases of chronic cystic mastitis that responded to neutralizing with good to excellent results.

INFLUENZA

Many of us have adopted a technique for relieving the acute symptoms of influenze (flu) virus infections which was developed by Dr. Miller. Neutralizing doses are prepared from regular influenza vaccine in the usual manner by making a series of dilutions of the same flu-preventing vaccine that your physician would administer in order to immunize you—the material used when "flu shots" are given. By testing and careful observation, a physician can often determine the specific dilution of this vaccine needed by each patient to reduce or completely clear the often severe discomfort and fever caused by an influenza infection.

Dr. Miller has told me that many of his patients have had their illness completely stopped when he gave them from one to three neutralizing doses a day for one to three days—the illness simply vanished.

MUMPS

Dr. Miller is certain that the limited number of cases of mumps he has treated have been benefited. The painful swelling in the side of the face was controlled within ten to thirty minutes after a treatment, and when the effects of the neutralizing dose wore off, four to eight hours later, and the pains returned, the symptoms were again relieved in a similar fashion by an additional neutralizing dose of the mumps vaccine.

HERPES

We do not know why Dr. Miller's technique for neutralizing with influenza virus vaccine has a beneficial effect on cases of shingles or other forms of herpes infection because the influenza virus and the herpes virus are not known to be closely related to each other. But many women with severe discomfort and badly inflamed genitals who were incapacitated by a genital infection with the herpes virus have had great relief and control of their illness with influenza neutralization. This work has been repeated by several of Dr. Miller's colleagues, including Dr. Firouz Farahmand of Portage, Indiana, a student of Dr. Miller's. Dr. Farahmand has seen seventy-two cases of herpes zoster (shingles) and used the neutralizing techniques on all of them. Among the seventy-two were four patients who came to him with pain that persisted after the infection itself had cleared. This was called a posteruption pain: The herpes zoster of the skin, the disease proper, had healed—there was nothing visible left on the skin, no fever, no illness—but the nerve pain persisted. All four of those patients improved on neutralizing technique. The terribly painful sensitivity of the skin on touch

or mild pressure (hyperesthesia), was either eliminated completely or greatly reduced in all patients, and this alone would
be a blessing because of the severe pain that goes on and on in
this illness.

Another colleague, Dr. Doris Rapp of Buffalo, recently reported on her similar experience with herpes and neutralization at the annual congress of the American College of Allergists.

CHICKEN POX

The chicken pox virus is a very close relative of the herpes
virus—indeed, it is thought by some experts in virus illness to
be the same disorder. (When I practiced pediatrics in the 1950s,
I was impressed by the fact that one member of a family had
a large patch of herpes eruption on her upper back and her
younger brother had chicken pox.) Dr. Miller recently told me
of four cases of chicken pox in which the children experienced
definite relief twenty minutes to a half hour after a neutralizing
dose of flu vaccine was administered, but he also emphasized
the fact that this was a clinical impression and that there were
so few cases that it was not possible for him to draw any conclusions. Dr. Miller feels strongly that exploration in this area must
be continued and enlarged because chicken pox, although it is
a minor disease of childhood, has caused fatal pneumonia and
fatal encephalitis. In some individuals whose immunity mechanisms were severely interfered with because of anticancer
treatment, chicken pox has led to fatalities.

The virus of infectious mononucleosis is not believed to be in
any way related to the influenza virus either, and again caution-
ing that his observations have been very limited, Dr. Miller
expressed the belief that the few patients he did treat were
benefited. He recognizes that the most that he, as a conscientious physician, can say is that this is another promising area
worth much additional investigation. Some day, an unimmu-
nized child critically ill with measles, polio, diphtheria, rabies,
or perhaps tetanus may be saved by a form of Dr. Miller's
development of Carleton Lee's neutralizing therapy.

PSORIASIS

An additional application of the neutralizing technique was developed for cases of psoriasis by Dr. Lee. He prepared solutions from the scales removed from patients suffering from psoriasis, prepared a patient-specific extract for each person and then a series of dilutions of the extract for each individual patient. In searching for the neutralizing dose in these patients, he noted that the wrong dilution of psoriasis scale extract would produce a flare-up of increased itching in this skin disease. When the proper individualized dose of this material was determined, the itching usually was completely relieved and many of the patients were actually cured of this very difficult to treat form of chronic dermatitis.

HYPERTENSION

There are an estimated twenty-five million cases of high blood pressure in this country that can have serious consequences. Dr. George Fricke, of Sacramento, California, has studied a group of twelve hypertensive patients employing fasting on spring water in a controlled environment. Dr. Ficke reported that nine of these patients (75 percent) responded completely, with their blood pressure returning to normal from levels as high as 210/140. In each of these cases the elimination of test-identified foods made it possible to discontinue previously required medications.

Only time will tell us what future research will uncover, and what important contributions will be made within the next few years. One thing is certain—we are going in the right direction. Bio-ecologic illness and allergy are at the core of many of the most serious threats to mankind's mental and physical well-being. Just knowing this is enough to change the course of medicine and the quality of health of every man, woman, and child.

Appendix: Instructions for Food-Allergy Testing

How to Begin Test Diets

It is best to begin by fasting for five days, but if you are not able to fast, you must avoid the foods in this diet in all forms (this means reading the labels on packages) for at least five days. It is necessary for your body to become free of the residual effects of the foods that will be eaten during the test. If you do not take this important first step, you will not have diagnostically reliable reactions to the foods as test meals. (At this time you might also begin the environmental control suggestions in chapter 6.)

If possible, purchase your foods from a health-food store so it will be as free as possible of insecticides, herbicides, color, preservatives, and waxes. Food, preferably, should be fresh. If not fresh, it should be frozen or canned-in-glass and not have *any* additional ingredients such as sugar because additional ingredients will interfere with testing. *Read the list of ingredients on the labels.* Food should not be wrapped in heat-sealed plastic packages because the food will absorb some chemical fumes from heated plastic wrap.

All mollusks, crustaceans, amphibians, fish, reptiles, and mammals should be broiled, baked, roasted, or steamed. Eggs may be poached in spring water or soft- or hard-boiled. Vegetables and fruits should be eaten raw, lightly steamed, boiled, baked or stir-fried.* Orange juice or grapefruit juice should be freshly squeezed at home or should be bottled in glass. It should

*Only if the oil being used has been tested and you did not react.

not be reconstituted from concentrate. Bananas should be purchased green and allowed to ripen at home for three to four days. Fruits should not be packed in syrup.

Do not use pepper, ketchup, mustard, sugar, honey, lemon or vinegar, etc., on any food.

Sea salt prepared by evaporation of clean sea water is permissible in limited amounts.

Spices can be tested by using them on test-negative foods. Oils can be tested by cooking test-negative foods in them, using them on test-negative foods as a "butter," or using them as a salad dressing on test-negative foods.

Nuts should be new and unprocessed.

Cereals should be boiled in spring water.

To test wheat, it is preferable to test it baked, puffed, and in boiled forms. Therefore, test matzoh, puffed wheat, and Ralston or Wheatena (boiled in spring water). Add salt.

To test rye buy rye crackers (no yeast).

To test barley buy barley *and* malt (malt is just toasted barley sprouts), boil the barley in spring water and add the malt.

To test oats eat oatmeal boiled in spring water and dry puffed oats.

To test cane sugar place two tablespoons of sugar into a glass of spring water. Stir well.

To test chocolate eat baker's chocolate or grate two to three one-ounce squares into a glass of ice cold spring water or into a fruit juice *if* you tested the juice and did not react.

To test baker's yeast, empty one packet of Red Star or its equivalent into a glass of ice cold spring water or into a fruit juice *if* you tested the juice and did not react.

To test brewer's yeast get some from the health-food store and mix one tablespoon into a glass of ice cold spring water or into fruit juice *if* you tested the juice and did not react.

To test food coloring, place three drops under the tongue.

How Much to Eat

Eat enough at one ten-to-fifteen-minute sitting to fill you up; don't eat for any longer than twenty minutes. The size portion for testing purposes is from two to four times the amount that is customarily eaten when the food is taken along with other foods at regular meals. Stop eating after twenty minutes.

Drink only spring water from glass bottles because there can be a problem even with spring water if it is bottled in plastic containers; chemicals that are present in the plastic may pass into the water. You may drink as much water as your thirst dictates but please do your best to take at least two quarts (eight glasses) a day. If you have need for salt on your food, you may add sea salt prepared from evaporated clean sea water to satisfy this need.

What to Expect

Some patients will react before they have finished eating; with others, it may take about twenty minutes before they begin to experience their first symptoms. Reactions usually start within the hour, but sometimes it is longer before symptoms appear; most reactions occur within four hours after eating. Delayed symptoms like muscle and joint pains or hives may occur eight to eighteen hours later, but this does not happen very often.

Make Notes about Your Reactions

Throughout the test period, write down the time you eat each food and any reactions that follow. Try writing your name, a series of numbers from 1 to 10, and an additional line or two such as your home address or a favorite quotation at ten-minute intervals to see if there are any changes in your handwriting. Handwriting changes are one of the indications of a nervous system reaction. It is not unusual for penmanship to change in quality and it may even become illegible. At times some letters and numbers are written backwards, errors in spelling occur, and as the reaction clears, penmanship returns to normal. Allergic changes of this type often occur in children with learning disabilities.

Reading is another excellent way to test some of your nervous system functions. Visual changes such as blurring and double vision are not uncommon, and while reading it is easy for you to detect changes in your ability to concentrate and to comprehend the material before you. Similar allergic reactions are produced in learning disabled children.

You should have some sodium bicarbonate (Arm and Hammer baking soda from the grocery store is fine) and some potassium bicarbonate (usually available as a loose powder at your pharmacy) on hand. It is best to let the reaction run its course to observe exactly what each food can do to you—whether you will have multiple symptoms or only one—but if your food reaction makes you very uncomfortable and you wish to stop it, do the following:

Mix 2 level tablespoons baking soda and 1 level tablespoon potassium bicarbonate thoroughly by shaking and turning them in a 4- to 6-ounce bottle. Put a heaping teaspoon of these mixed bicarbonates in 16 ounces of water, and drink it down as quickly as possible—it will taste quite salty. Your reaction should cease in a matter of minutes as these alkaline salts temporarily change your body chemistry by eliminating the local acids that accumulate where reactions are occurring. This mixture of alkaline salts should not be taken by individuals who have heart or kidney disease unless their physician authorizes them to do so.

If you have Alka Seltzer Gold on hand, take two tablets with two glasses of water: one tablet in each 8-ounce glass. Do not take the regular Alka Seltzer—it contains aspirin. If you read the Alka Seltzer Gold label, you'll see it contains sodium bicarbonate and potassium bicarbonate with a few other ingredients. It works quite well, but for some people not as well as the mixture of sodium and potassium bicarbonates that you can prepare yourself.

(See chapter 8 for a complete discussion of temporarily relieving allergic symptoms due to food and chemicals in food.)

WARNING: If you have addictive food allergy it is possible that your withdrawal symptoms may make you quite uncomfortable as the manifestations of your usual disorder flare up during this period. Remember that the withdrawal phase is followed in most instances by a period of increased sensitivity to offending foods. A disorder that has been completely or partially submerged now is capable of causing acute flare-ups of considerable intensity. People with physical and mental problems who have required hospitalization for these specific disorders *should not follow this diet without professional supervision.*

If you have severe asthma, epilepsy, diabetes, or severe depression, you should not risk undergoing the increased intensity of symptoms that are associated with the withdrawal phase or the increased severity of reactions that might be evoked by individual foods in the five-day diet. A good rule of thumb would be: When in doubt, do not become involved in this program without the supervision of a physician with training and experience in bio-ecologic disorders.

Index